I0841296

OPTIMAL NUTRITION

UNDERSTANDING THE MICROBIOME TO IMPROVE OUR HEALTH

DAVID SANDUA

*"The right balance of nutritious foods
is essential for optimal functioning of mind and body."*

Deepak Chopra

INDEX

I. INTRODUCTION

There has been a growing interest in the field of microbiology, particularly in understanding the microbiome and its impact on human health. The microbiome refers to the complex community of microorganisms that reside in and on the human body, primarily in the gastrointestinal tract. These microorganisms play a crucial role in maintaining the overall health and well-being of an individual. They aid in the digestion and absorption of nutrients, produce essential vitamins, and interact with the immune system. Emerging research has shown that the foods we consume have a direct influence on the composition and function of our microbiomes. This recognition of the relationship between nutrition and the microbiome has given rise to the concept of optimal nutrition, which emphasizes the consumption of certain foods to support a healthy microbiome and improve overall health. By delving into the science of the microbiome and exploring the concept of optimal nutrition, we can gain valuable insights into how our dietary choices affect our microbiomes and subsequently impact our holistic wellness.

The microbiome is a vast collection of microorganisms, including bacteria, viruses, fungi, and archaea, that play a crucial role in the maintenance of human health. These microorganisms not only outnumber our own cells but also carry three million genes, collectively known as the microbiome genome, a number exceeding our own genome by a factor of 150. The microbiome is a dynamic ecosystem that evolves throughout an individual's lifespan. It begins to shape shortly after birth and continues to develop and diversify over time, influenced by various factors such as genetics, the environment, and, importantly, diet. Understanding the composition and function of the microbiome has been a significant area of research, as scientists are looking to harness its potential for the development of personalized therapies and interventions. By investigating the intricate relationship between host genetics, the microbiome, and various health outcomes, researchers aim to unravel the mechanisms through which the microbiome impacts an individual's health.

One of the key factors influencing the composition and function of the microbiome is the diet. Modern dietary patterns have shifted towards processed foods, high in refined carbohydrates, unhealthy fats, and additives. These dietary patterns have been associated with an altered microbiome composition, characterized by a decrease in beneficial microbes and an overgrowth of potentially harmful ones. Conversely, diets rich in whole, unprocessed foods, such as fruits, vegetables, whole grains, and lean proteins, have been shown to support a diverse and thriving microbiome. The beneficial bacteria in the gut thrive on fiber, found abundantly in these unprocessed foods. This symbiotic relationship between the microbiome and our dietary choices unveils the potential for improving our health through optimal nutrition, which involves consuming foods that support the growth and balance of beneficial bacteria in our microbiomes.

Optimal nutrition emphasizes the inclusion of foods that nourish and support the microbiome, ultimately promoting overall health and well-being. Certain types of dietary fiber, known as prebiotic fiber, serve as a source of nutrition for the beneficial bacteria in the gut. By consuming prebiotic-rich foods, such as fruits, vegetables, legumes, and whole grains, we can foster the growth of these beneficial microbes and improve the diversity of our microbiome. Probiotics, which are live bacteria and yeasts, have been shown to confer health benefits when consumed as supplements or in fermented foods. Probiotic-rich foods like yogurt, kefir, sauerkraut, and kimchi can help introduce beneficial bacteria into the gut, supporting a healthy microbiome.

The impact of the microbiome on human health is far-reaching, extending beyond digestion and nutrient absorption. Research has linked alterations in the microbiome to various health conditions, including obesity, diabetes, inflammatory bowel disease, allergies, and even mental health disorders like depression and anxiety. By understanding the intricate interplay between the microbiome and nutrition, we can harness this knowledge to optimize our dietary choices for holistic wellness. It is an exciting field of study that holds great potential for personalized medicine and prevention strategies, by tailoring diets based on an individual's microbiome composition.

Understanding the science of the microbiome and the influence of nutrition on its composition and function is crucial for improving our overall health. The microbiome, a dynamic and complex ecosystem, plays a vital role in numerous physiological processes. Optimal nutrition, through the consumption of prebiotic and probiotic-rich foods, supports a thriving microbiome and may contribute to a range of health benefits. By exploring the interplay between the microbiome and nutrition, we can gain valuable insights into how our dietary choices influence our microbiomes and subsequently impact our holistic wellness. As research in this field progresses, it holds tremendous promise for personalized approaches to healthcare and disease prevention.

DEFINITION OF THE MICROBIOME AND ITS IMPORTANCE IN HUMAN HEALTH

The microbiome refers to the collection of microorganisms, including bacteria, fungi, viruses, and other microbes, that inhabit the human body. These microorganisms reside in various regions of the body, such as the skin, mouth, and gut, forming a complex ecosystem that interacts with our physiology and plays a crucial role in maintaining our health. The significance of the microbiome in human health is now widely recognized, with emerging research shedding light on its involvement in various aspects of our well-being, including digestion, immune function, and disease prevention. The human gut microbiome, in particular, has garnered significant attention due to its vital role in digestion and overall metabolism. It consists of trillions of microbes that coexist with our own cells, working together symbiotically to break down complex carbohydrates, produce essential vitamins, and produce short-chain fatty acids, which provide an energy source for our cells. This intricate interaction between the gut microbiome and our diet is central to our ability to extract the full nutritional value from the foods we consume.

The gut microbiome also plays a crucial role in regulating our immune function. The presence of certain strains of bacteria in the gut helps in the development and maturation of our immune system, allowing it to distinguish between harmful pathogens and harmless substances. This process, called immune tolerance, helps prevent an immune response to harmless substances such as food or commensal bacteria, reducing the risk of allergies and autoimmune diseases.

In addition to digestion and immune function, the microbiome has been implicated in various other aspects of human health. For instance, recent studies have shown that alterations in the composition of the gut microbiome may contribute to the development of chronic diseases, including obesity, type 2 diabetes, and cardiovascular diseases. The diversity and balance of the gut microbiome appear to be crucial in maintaining metabolic homeostasis, with dysbiosis, a disruption in the gut microbial community, being associated with metabolic disorders.

The microbial ecosystem that exists on our skin has also been found to contribute to human health. The skin microbiome, populated by numerous species of bacteria, fungi, and viruses, forms a protective barrier against pathogens, preventing their colonization and reducing the risk of infections. Research has shown that the composition of the skin microbiome influences the skin's immune response and contributes to maintaining the integrity of our skin barrier. Imbalances in the skin microbiome may lead to various skin conditions, such as acne, eczema, and psoriasis, highlighting the importance of maintaining a healthy microbial community on our skin. The oral microbiome, consisting of various microorganisms residing in the mouth, also plays a vital role in human health. These microbes contribute to the breakdown of food particles, promoting efficient digestion and nutrient absorption. They contribute to maintaining oral health by preventing the overgrowth of harmful bacteria that can cause dental caries and gum diseases. The oral microbiome has even been linked to systemic health, with evidence suggesting that dysbiosis in the mouth may contribute to the development of cardiovascular diseases and respiratory infections.

Given the significant impact of the microbiome on human health, understanding its composition and function has become a crucial area of research. Recent advancements in sequencing technologies have enabled researchers to study the microbiome in greater detail and gain insight into its complex interactions with our body. This knowledge has paved the way for potential therapeutic interventions aimed at modulating the microbiome to improve human health. Probiotics, live microorganisms that can confer health benefits when consumed, have gained popularity as a means of promoting a healthy microbiome. These supplements contain specific strains of bacteria or yeasts that have been shown to positively impact various aspects of human health. Prebiotics, on the other hand, are indigestible dietary fibers that selectively stimulate the growth and activity of beneficial bacteria in the gut. By incorporating these components into our diet, we can potentially support the growth of beneficial microorganisms and restore balance within our microbiome.

The microbiome is a collection of microorganisms that reside in various regions of the human body, including the gut, skin, and mouth. Its importance in human health cannot be overstated, as it is involved in diverse functions such as digestion, immune function, and disease prevention. The gut microbiome, in particular, plays a crucial role in extracting nutrients from our diet and maintaining metabolic homeostasis. Imbalances in the gut microbiome have been associated with various chronic diseases. Similarly, the skin and oral microbiomes contribute to maintaining the integrity of their respective barriers and preventing infections. Understanding the composition and function of the microbiome has opened avenues for potential therapeutic interventions aimed at modulating its dynamics to improve human

health. By harnessing the power of the microbiome, we can optimize our nutrition and pave the way for holistic wellness.

THE RELATIONSHIP BETWEEN THE MICROBIOME AND NUTRITION

One of the key aspects of understanding the microbiome and its impact on human health is exploring the relationship between the microbiome and nutrition. The microbiome, which consists of trillions of microorganisms living in and on our bodies, plays a crucial role in nutrient metabolism and absorption. These micro-organisms have been found to have a significant influence on various health outcomes, including immune function, mental health, and metabolism. Nutrition, on the other hand, refers to the intake of food and how our bodies utilize the essential nutrients present in these foods. The interaction between the micro-biome and nutrition is a complex and bidirectional relationship, where the composition and function of the microbiome can be influenced by our dietary choices, and, in turn, the microbiome can impact nutrient availability and metabolism.

One way in which the microbiome and nutrition are intercon-nected is through the fermentation of dietary fibers by our gut bacteria. Dietary fibers, which are primarily found in plant-based foods such as fruits, vegetables, whole grains, and leg-umes, are indigestible by humans. Our gut microbes have the ability to break down these fibers through fermentation, pro-ducing short-chain fatty acids (SCFAs) as byproducts. SCFAs, such as butyrate, propionate, and acetate, have been shown to have numerous health benefits. They serve as an energy source for the cells lining our gut, promote the growth of beneficial bacteria, and have anti-inflammatory effects. SCFAs also have a positive impact on our metabolism, as they have been found to reduce the risk of obesity and metabolic disorders.

Another way in which the microbiome and nutrition interact is through the modulation of the gut-brain axis. This bidirectional communication system between the gut and the brain involves several signaling pathways, including the release of neuro-transmitters, hormones, and immune molecules. Emerging evidence suggests that the gut microbiome plays a crucial role in influencing our mood, behavior, and overall mental health. For example, certain strains of gut bacteria have been found to produce neurotransmitters such as serotonin and dopamine, which play key roles in regulating mood and emotions. Imbalances in the gut microbiome, known as dysbiosis, have been associated with mental health conditions such as depression and anxiety. The composition of the microbiome can also impact nutrient availability and metabolism. Our gut bacteria, for instance, can produce enzymes that aid in the digestion and absorption of certain nutrients. Studies have shown that specific bacteria can break down complex carbohydrates, proteins, and fats into simpler forms that our bodies can absorb and utilize. In addition, the presence of certain bacteria can also influence the bioavailability of various vitamins and minerals. For example, some gut bacteria produce enzymes that convert dietary compounds into their active forms, allowing our bodies to efficiently metabolize essential nutrients like vitamin K and vitamin B12.

Conversely, the types of foods we consume can shape the diversity and function of our gut microbiome. A diet rich in plant-based foods, for example, has been associated with a more diverse and beneficial microbial community. Plant-based diets provide a wide range of fibers, prebiotics, and phytochemicals that promote the growth of beneficial bacteria and contribute to a healthy microbiome. A diet high in processed foods, sugars, and unhealthy fats has been shown to negatively impact the diversity and function of the microbiome. These dietary choices can lead to dysbiosis, inflammation, and the overgrowth of harmful bacteria, increasing the risk of various diseases such as obesity, type 2 diabetes, and inflammatory bowel diseases. The relationship between the microbiome and nutrition is a complex and bidirectional one. The composition and function of the microbiome can be influenced by our dietary choices, while the microbiome, in turn, can impact nutrient availability and metabolism. Understanding this relationship is crucial for optimizing our nutrition and improving our overall health. By consuming a diverse and plant-based diet, we can promote the growth of beneficial bacteria in our gut, enhance nutrient absorption, and reduce the risk of various diseases. This knowledge highlights the importance of considering the microbiome when making dietary choices for holistic wellness. The relationship between our diet and our health is a complex one, influenced by an intricate network of interactions between our bodies and the trillions of microbes that inhabit our gastrointestinal tract, known as the microbiome. The microbiome is a diverse ecological community composed of bacteria, viruses, fungi, and other microorganisms, and it plays a crucial role in maintaining our health and well-being. Recent advances in scientific research have unveiled the intricate connections between our dietary choices, the composition of our microbiomes, and their impact on our overall health. By understanding the microbiome and the ways in which it is influenced by our diet, we can make informed decisions about optimal nutrition and pave the way for a healthier future.

When it comes to the microbiome, diversity is key. A healthy microbiome is characterized by a rich diversity of microorganisms, with a balance of beneficial bacteria that aid in digestion, nutrient absorption, and immune function. A disrupted microbiome, characterized by a loss of diversity and an overgrowth of harmful bacteria, has been linked to a range of health issues, including obesity, diabetes, and inflammatory bowel disease. Promoting a diverse microbiome should be a cornerstone of any dietary approach aimed at improving our health. One of the most effective ways to promote a diverse microbiome is through a plant-rich diet. Plant-based foods, such as fruits, vegetables, whole grains, legumes, and nuts, are rich in dietary fiber, which is indigestible by human enzymes but serves as a valuable food source for our gut bacteria. By consuming a diet that is high in fiber, we can promote the growth of beneficial bacteria in our gut, which are capable of fermenting this fiber, producing short-chain fatty acids (SCFAs), and reducing inflammation in the gut. In addition to promoting diversity, it is important to cultivate a healthy balance between different microbial species. Emerging evidence suggests that a diet high in saturated fats and added sugars can alter the composition of the microbiome, favoring the growth of harmful bacteria and impairing the function of beneficial ones. This dysbiosis, or imbalance, has been linked to a variety of chronic diseases, including obesity, insulin resistance, and cardiovascular disease. It is crucial to limit the consumption of high-fat, high-sugar foods and instead prioritize foods that support a healthy microbiome. The role of fermented foods in promoting a healthy microbiome should not be underestimated. Fermented foods, such as yogurt, sauerkraut, kefir, and kimchi, are rich in beneficial bacteria, known as probiotics, which can colonize our gut and contribute to its overall health. These probiotics help to restore and maintain the balance of our microbiome, improving digestion, nutrient absorption, and immune function. Incorporating fermented foods into our diet can thus be a simple and effective way to support our microbiome and optimize our health. It is not just about what we eat, but also how we eat that matters. Our eating patterns and habits can have a significant impact on our microbiome and our health. Research suggests that consuming smaller, more frequent meals throughout the day, as opposed to a few large meals, can promote a more stable and diverse microbiome. Mindful eating, or paying attention to the sensory experience of eating and being present in the moment, has been shown to improve digestion and nutrient absorption, as well as reduce stress and enhance overall well-being. By adopting healthier eating patterns and cultivating a mindful approach to food, we can support the health of our microbiome and improve our overall health and wellness. The science of the microbiome provides valuable insights into the intricate connections between our diet, our microbiomes, and our health. By understanding the role of the microbiome in maintaining our health and well-being, we can make informed choices about optimal nutrition and adopt dietary approaches that promote a diverse and balanced microbiome. Through a plant-rich diet, moderation in the consumption of high-fat, high-sugar foods, and the incorporation of fermented foods, we can support our microbiome and pave the way for holistic wellness. By cultivating healthier eating patterns and adopting a mindful approach to food, we can further enhance the health of our microbiome and improve our overall quality of life. This knowledge empowers us to take control of our own health and make proactive choices that can lead to a healthier and more fulfilling life.

THE VITAL CONNECTION: OPTIMAL NUTRITION AND THE MICROBIOME FOR HOLISTIC WELLNESS

The microbiome refers to the ecological community of microorganisms, including bacteria, fungi, viruses, and other microbes, that inhabit our bodies. While microorganisms may have been historically associated with disease, recent research has shed light on the largely beneficial role they play in supporting our overall health and well-being. In fact, the microbiome has been described as an "invisible organ" that is intricately involved in many physiological processes, including digestion, immune function, and even mental health. Understanding the science behind the microbiome and its impact on human health is crucial for developing optimal nutrition strategies that can enhance the diversity and balance of our microbial communities.

One of the key aspects to consider when it comes to the microbiome is its remarkable diversity. Each individual harbors a unique composition of microorganisms that is influenced by factors such as genetics, environment, and most importantly, diet. It is estimated that the average human microbiome is made up of trillions of microorganisms, many of which reside in our gastrointestinal tract, particularly the large intestine. This rich and complex ecosystem plays a crucial role in breaking down and absorbing nutrients from the foods we eat, as well as producing essential vitamins and other metabolites that contribute to our overall health. Not all microorganisms within the microbiome are beneficial. Imbalances in the composition of the microbiome, known as dysbiosis, have been associated with a range of health conditions, including inflammatory bowel diseases, obesity, and even mental illnesses such as depression and anxiety. This highlights the importance of promoting a healthy and diverse microbiome through optimal nutrition. So, how can we improve our microbiome through diet?

First and foremost, a diet that is rich in fiber is essential for nurturing a healthy microbiome. Fiber acts as a prebiotic, providing nourishment for beneficial bacteria in the gut. Foods that are high in fiber include fruits, vegetables, whole grains, legumes, and nuts. Consuming a variety of plant-based foods can help diversify the microbial ecosystem in our gut, promoting the growth of beneficial bacteria and enhancing the overall stability and resilience of the microbiome. In addition to fiber, fermented foods are another key component of a microbiome-friendly diet. Fermented foods, such as yogurt, sauerkraut, kimchi, and kefir, contain live bacteria and other microorganisms that can directly influence the composition of the microbiome. By consuming these foods regularly, we can introduce beneficial bacteria into our gut and support the growth of a healthy microbial community. Fermented foods have been shown to improve digestion, enhance nutrient absorption, and strengthen the immune system. It is important to note that not all fermented foods are created equal, and commercial products may vary in their probiotic content and efficacy. Choosing high-quality, traditionally prepared fermented foods or considering probiotic supplements may be beneficial. Another factor to consider in optimizing the microbiome is the reduction of processed and sugary foods. These types of foods have been shown to negatively impact the diversity and richness of the microbiome, favoring the growth of potentially harmful bacteria. Diets high in added sugars have been linked to an increased risk of chronic diseases, including obesity, type 2 diabetes, and cardiovascular diseases. By choosing whole, unprocessed foods and reducing our intake of added sugars, we can support the growth of beneficial bacteria and promote a healthy microbiome. It is important to acknowledge that the microbiome is a complex and evolving ecosystem that is still not fully understood. Research in this field is ongoing, and the recommendations presented here may evolve as more insights are gained. The evidence thus far supports the notion that a diverse and balanced microbiome is crucial for our overall health and well-being. Incorporating the principles of optimal nutrition, such as consuming a plant-based, fiber-rich diet and incorporating fermented foods, can help nurture a healthy microbiome and pave the way for improved physical and mental health. By understanding and harnessing the power of the microbiome, we can take proactive steps toward achieving holistic wellness. Optimal nutrition plays a crucial role in maintaining a healthy microbiome, which in turn has a profound impact on human health. The microbiome refers to the collection of microorganisms, including bacteria, fungi, and viruses, that reside in our body, particularly in our gut. This complex ecosystem, also known as the gut microbiota, plays an essential role in various physiological processes, such as digestion, immune function, and even mental health. Understanding the science behind the microbiome and its relationship to nutrition is key to achieving holistic wellness. Firstly, the gut microbiome is highly influenced by the foods we consume. Certain dietary components, such as fiber, promote the growth of beneficial bacteria in the gut. Fibrous foods, like fruits, vegetables, whole grains, and legumes, are rich sources of prebiotics, which serve as fuel for the beneficial bacteria. When the beneficial bacteria digest these prebiotics, they produce short-chain fatty acids (SCFAs), which have anti-inflammatory properties and contribute to overall gut health. Conversely, a low-fiber diet can lead to a decrease in the diversity and abundance of beneficial bacteria, resulting in an imbalanced microbiome and potential health issues.

The type of fats we consume also has an impact on the microbiome. A diet high in saturated fats, commonly found in processed foods, red meat, and full-fat dairy products, can alter the composition of gut bacteria and increase the levels of harmful bacteria. These harmful bacteria produce metabolites that contribute to chronic inflammation, a known risk factor for various diseases, including cardiovascular disease and obesity. Incorporating healthier fats, such as those found in nuts, seeds, oily fish, and olive oil, can enhance the diversity of the gut microbiota and promote a more balanced microbiome.

In addition to fiber and fats, the role of protein in the microbiome cannot be understated. Animal-based protein sources, such as meat and dairy, can lead to an increase in the production of harmful metabolites, such as trimethylamine N-oxide (TMAO), which has been implicated in cardiovascular disease. Conversely, plant-based protein sources, like legumes, nuts, and seeds, promote the growth of beneficial bacteria, and their digestion produces health-promoting metabolites. Incorporating more plant-based proteins into the diet is not only beneficial for human health but also for maintaining a healthy microbiome.

The impact of processed and ultra-processed foods on the microbiome cannot be ignored. These foods, typically high in added sugars, unhealthy fats, and artificial additives, not only lack essential nutrients but also disrupt the delicate balance of the gut microbiota. For instance, excessive consumption of added sugars can lead to an overgrowth of harmful bacteria, which has been linked to obesity and metabolic disorders. By contrast, a diet rich in whole, unprocessed foods provides the necessary nutrients for the growth of beneficial bacteria and supports a healthier microbiome. The scientific community has increasingly recognized the importance of the gut-brain axis, which refers to the bidirectional communication between the gut and the brain. Emerging evidence suggests that the microbiome plays a role in mental health and brain function. Studies have shown that a disturbed gut microbiome, often as a result of an unhealthy diet, is associated with an increased risk of mental health disorders, such as depression and anxiety. A healthy microbiome, supported by optimal nutrition, can contribute to improved cognitive function and overall mental well-being. Optimal nutrition and the microbiome are intricately connected for holistic wellness. The foods we eat influence the composition and function of our gut microbiota, which, in turn, impacts various aspects of our health. Incorporating a diet rich in fiber, healthy fats, and plant-based proteins can promote a diverse and balanced microbiome, reducing the risk of chronic diseases and supporting optimal physical and mental well-being. Minimizing the consumption of processed and ultra-processed foods is vital for maintaining a healthy microbiome. By understanding and leveraging the science of the microbiome, we can take proactive steps towards improving our health and achieving holistic wellness.

II. THE SCIENCE OF THE MICROBIOME

The human microbiome is a complex and fascinating ecosystem consisting of trillions of microorganisms, such as bacteria, viruses, fungi, and other microbes. These microbes reside in various parts of our bodies, including the skin, mouth, and most notably, the gastrointestinal tract. The science of the microbiome revolves around understanding the composition, diversity, and functionality of these microorganisms, as well as their intricate interactions with our bodies. Over the past decade, significant advancements have been made in this field, unraveling the profound impact of the microbiome on our overall health and well-being. The gastrointestinal tract is the primary site where the microbiome exerts its influence. The gut microbiome plays a crucial role in digestion, nutrient absorption, and the synthesis of essential vitamins and metabolites. Certain bacteria in the gut, such as Bacteroidetes and Firmicutes, aid in breaking down complex carbohydrates that are otherwise indigestible by our bodies. They produce enzymes that degrade these complex molecules into simpler forms, allowing us to absorb the nutrients efficiently. The gut microbiome plays a vital role in the maturation and development of our immune system. The presence of specific microbes stimulates the immune system to enhance its responses to external pathogens. Conversely, an imbalance in the gut microbiome, known as dysbiosis, can lead to immune dysfunction, increasing the risk of autoimmune diseases, allergies, and infections. Research has also shown that the gut microbiome has a profound impact on our mental health and brain function. The gut-brain axis is a bidirectional communication system between the gut and the brain, facilitated by the microbiome. Certain bacteria produce neurotransmitters, such as serotonin and dopamine, which are essential for mood regulation. Imbalances in the gut microbiome have been linked to various mental health disorders, including anxiety, depression, and even neurodegenerative diseases like Alzheimer's.

In addition to these impacts, the gut microbiome also influences our metabolism and body weight. Recent studies have demonstrated that certain species of bacteria are associated with obesity, while others are associated with leanness. The composition of the gut microbiome can affect the breakdown and absorption of dietary fats, ultimately influencing energy storage and expenditure. The gut microbiome can affect the production of hormones that regulate hunger and satiety, such as leptin and ghrelin, further impacting our eating behaviors and body weight. Understanding the science behind the microbiome has profound implications for improving our health and well-being. While genetics play a role in determining the composition of our microbiome, it is highly influenced by environmental factors, particularly our diet. The foods we eat directly impact the diversity and abundance of the microorganisms in our gut. Diets rich in fiber, prebiotics, and fermented foods promote the growth of beneficial bacteria, leading to a more diverse and balanced microbiome. Diets high in processed foods, added sugars, and unhealthy fats promote the growth of harmful bacteria, leading to dysbiosis and an increased risk of various diseases. The overuse of antibiotics, which indiscriminately kill both harmful and beneficial bacteria, can disrupt the delicate balance of the gut microbiome, leading to long-term consequences on our health. To optimize our nutrition and promote a healthy microbiome, a holistic approach is required. It is essential to consume a diverse range of plant-based foods, including fruits, vegetables, whole grains, and legumes, which provide a rich source of fiber, phytochemicals, and other essential nutrients. These foods act as prebiotics, serving as a fuel source for the beneficial bacteria in our gut. Incorporating fermented foods, such as yogurt, kefir, sauerkraut, and kimchi, can introduce beneficial strains of bacteria into our gut. These probiotics can help restore the balance of the microbiome and promote overall gut health. Reducing the consumption of processed foods, refined sugars, and unhealthy fats can prevent dysbiosis and the negative consequences associated with it. The science of the microbiome has significantly expanded our understanding of the complex relationships between our bodies and the trillions of microorganisms that inhabit our gut. The microbiome plays a vital role in digestion, immune function, brain health, metabolism, and overall well-being. By understanding the impacts of our diet on the microbiome, we can make informed choices about what we eat, optimizing our nutrition, and improving our health holistically. The future of medicine lies in unlocking the potential of the microbiome and harnessing its power to address various health conditions and promote wellness.

THE COMPOSITION AND DIVERSITY OF THE MICROBIOME

The composition and diversity of the microbiome, specifically the gut microbiome, play a critical role in maintaining our overall health. As mentioned earlier, the gut microbiome is composed of trillions of microorganisms, including bacteria, viruses, fungi, and other microbes. While bacterial cells outnumber human cells in our bodies, the specific composition of the gut microbiome can vary greatly among individuals. This diversity is influenced by various factors, including genetics, diet, lifestyle, and environmental exposures. The first factor contributing to the composition of the gut microbiome is genetics. Research has shown that genetics can influence the types of microorganisms present in the gut. Each individual has a unique set of genes that influence the development and function of the gut microbiome. Genetic variations can affect the abundance and diversity of certain bacterial species in the gut. For example, studies have identified specific genes that are associated with the presence of certain beneficial bacteria, such as Bifidobacterium and Lactobacillus, which are known to have health-promoting effects. Understanding the genetic factors that shape the gut microbiome can help us identify individuals who may be more prone to certain health conditions and develop personalized interventions to improve their gut health. Another important factor in the composition of the gut microbiome is diet. The foods we eat directly influence the types of bacteria that thrive in our gut. Certain dietary components, such as fiber, act as prebiotics, providing a food source for beneficial bacteria. When we consume fiber-rich foods, such as fruits, vegetables, and whole grains, these prebiotics reach the colon undigested, where they are fermented by bacteria. This fermentation process produces short-chain fatty acids, such as butyrate, which are essential for maintaining a healthy gut environment. Diets high in processed foods and low in fiber can lead to a decrease in the abundance of beneficial bacteria and an increase in potentially harmful bacteria. A diet rich in fiber promotes a diverse and balanced microbiome, which is associated with improved immune function, metabolism, and mental health. In addition to genetics and diet, lifestyle factors also influence the composition and diversity of the gut microbiome. For example, stress can alter the gut microbiome by affecting the production of stress hormones, such as cortisol. Chronic stress can lead to an imbalance in the gut microbiome, with a decrease in beneficial bacteria and an increase in pathogenic bacteria. Regular physical activity has been shown to have a positive impact on the gut microbiome, promoting the growth of beneficial bacteria and reducing inflammation. Sleep patterns also influence the gut microbiome, with disruption in sleep leading to changes in the composition of bacteria. Environmental exposures, such as antibiotics and other medications, can disrupt the gut microbiome by killing off both harmful and beneficial bacteria. It is important to note that while antibiotics can be life-saving in certain situations, their overuse or misuse can have detrimental effects on the gut microbiome. It is crucial to use antibiotics judiciously and consider strategies to restore and maintain a healthy gut microbiome following their use. The composition and diversity of the microbiome, specifically the gut microbiome, are influenced by a multitude of factors, including genetics, diet, lifestyle, and environmental exposures. Each individual has a unique set of microorganisms in their gut, which can have profound effects on their overall health. Understanding the factors that shape the gut microbiome can help us develop strategies to optimize its composition for improved health outcomes. Further research is needed to unravel the complex interactions between the microbiome and various aspects of human health, paving the way for personalized approaches to nutrition and healthcare that take into account our individual microbiome profiles. By harnessing the power of the microbiome, we can work towards achieving optimal nutrition and holistic wellness.

THE ROLE OF THE MICROBIOME IN DIGESTION AND METABOLISM

The role of the microbiome in digestion and metabolism is complex and multi-faceted. One of the key functions of the microbiome is the breakdown of dietary fiber. Human enzymes are unable to fully digest fiber, but certain bacteria in the gut, known as fiber degraders, have the ability to break down these complex carbohydrates into smaller molecules that can be absorbed by the body. This process, known as fermentation, produces short-chain fatty acids (SCFAs), such as acetate, propionate, and butyrate, which are important sources of energy for the cells that line the colon. SCFAs also play a role in regulating satiety and appetite, as well as glucose and lipid metabolism.

Research has shown that alterations in the composition of the gut microbiome can have a significant impact on metabolic health. For example, a dysbiotic microbiome, characterized by an imbalance of harmful bacteria, has been associated with insulin resistance and obesity. This is thought to occur through the production of molecules called lipopolysaccharides (LPS) by certain bacteria in the gut. LPS can trigger chronic low-grade inflammation, which has been implicated in the development of insulin resistance and metabolic disorders. Dysbiosis can lead to increased production of secondary bile acids, which have been shown to promote the accumulation of fat in the liver and contribute to the development of non-alcoholic fatty liver disease (NAFLD). A diverse and balanced gut microbiome can support optimal digestion and metabolism. Research has shown that certain beneficial bacteria, such as Bacteroides and Akkermansia muciniphila, are associated with improved metabolic health. These bacteria have been shown to enhance the production of SCFAs and improve gut barrier function, which can help reduce inflammation and improve insulin sensitivity. A diverse gut microbiome has been associated with a lower risk of obesity and metabolic syndrome. It is important to note that the composition of the gut microbiome is not solely determined by genetics, but is also influenced by diet and lifestyle factors. A diet high in fiber and plant-based foods has been shown to promote the growth of beneficial bacteria and increase microbial diversity. This is attributed to the fact that fiber-rich foods serve as a fuel source for fiber degraders. In contrast, a diet high in processed foods and saturated fats has been associated with a less diverse and less healthy microbiome. Interestingly, recent research has also highlighted the role of the microbiome in the metabolism of certain dietary nutrients. For example, the microbiome has been shown to influence the absorption and metabolism of dietary fats. Specific bacteria, such as Bacteroides and Firmicutes, have been implicated in the conversion of dietary fats into bioactive compounds, such as short-chain fatty acids and secondary bile acids. These compounds can have both beneficial and detrimental effects on health, depending on their concentration and the overall composition of the microbiome. The microbiome plays a critical role in digestion and metabolism. The breakdown of dietary fiber by fiber degraders produces short-chain fatty acids, which are important sources of energy for the body. A dysbiotic microbiome can contribute to metabolic disorders, such as obesity and insulin resistance, through the production of pro-inflammatory molecules and alterations in bile acid metabolism. A diverse and balanced gut microbiome is associated with improved metabolic health. Diet and lifestyle factors, such as fiber intake and the consumption of plant-based foods, play a key role in shaping the composition of the gut microbiome. Future research in this field holds promise for developing targeted interventions to improve digestion and metabolism through modulation of the microbiome.

THE FACTORS THAT INFLUENCE THE DEVELOPMENT AND MAINTENANCE OF A HEALTHY MICROBIOME

One of the key factors that influences the development and maintenance of a healthy microbiome is diet. The foods we consume play a crucial role in shaping the composition and diversity of our gut microbiota. A diet that is rich in fiber and plant-based foods has been linked to a more diverse and robust microbiome. Fiber acts as a prebiotic, providing nourishment for the beneficial bacteria in our gut. It is broken down by these bacteria into short-chain fatty acids, which have numerous health benefits, including reducing inflammation and improving gut barrier function. A diet high in processed foods, sugar, and saturated fats has been associated with a less diverse microbiome and an overgrowth of harmful bacteria. These unhealthy dietary choices can lead to various health conditions, including obesity, insulin resistance, and chronic inflammation. Adopting a balanced and nutrient-dense diet that includes a variety of plant-based foods is crucial for promoting a healthy microbiome. There has been a growing interest in understanding the intricate interactions between our bodies and the trillions of microorganisms that reside within us, known as the microbiome. The microbiome, especially the gut microbiome, plays a crucial role in our overall health and well-being. It is a complex ecosystem that consists of billions of bacteria, fungi, viruses, and other microorganisms that live in symbiosis with us. These microorganisms have co-evolved with us over millions of years, and they perform a multitude of essential functions that contribute to our overall health. From aiding in digestion and nutrient absorption to modulating our immune system, the microbiome has a profound impact on our overall well-being.

One of the critical factors that influence the composition and function of our microbiome is the food we eat. Our diets can either promote the growth of beneficial bacteria or contribute to the proliferation of harmful ones. Unhealthy diets rich in processed foods, sugar, and saturated fats can negatively impact the diversity and stability of our microbiome. It can lead to a decrease in beneficial bacteria and an increase in harmful bacteria, leading to various health issues such as obesity, diabetes, and inflammatory bowel disease. A healthy diet rich in fruits, vegetables, whole grains, and fiber promotes a diverse and stable microbiome. These foods contain essential nutrients and prebiotics that act as fuel for the beneficial bacteria in our gut, promoting their growth and enhancing their functions. One of the key nutrients that play a crucial role in supporting a healthy microbiome is fiber. Fiber is a type of carbohydrate that cannot be digested by our bodies, but it serves as an important source of food for our gut bacteria. When we consume dietary fiber, it passes through our digestive system largely intact, reaching the colon where our gut bacteria reside. The fiber acts as a prebiotic, nourishing the beneficial bacteria and promoting their growth. As the beneficial bacteria digest the fiber, they produce short-chain fatty acids (SCFAs) as byproducts. SCFAs are crucial for gut health as they provide energy to the cells lining our colon, reduce inflammation, and regulate our immune system. In addition to fiber, other prebiotics such as resistant starch and oligosaccharides also serve as food for our gut bacteria, promoting their growth and enhancing their functions. Probiotics, another important component of the microbiome, also play a key role in supporting our overall health. Probiotics are live microorganisms that, when consumed in adequate quantities, confer health benefits to the host. They help in maintaining the balance of our gut microbiome by crowding out harmful bacteria and promoting the growth of beneficial ones. Probiotics can be found naturally in fermented foods such as yogurt, kefir, sauerkraut, and kimchi. They can also be consumed in the form of supplements. Research has shown that probiotics can help in alleviating symptoms of digestive disorders such as irritable bowel syndrome and inflammatory bowel disease. They have also been found to support our immune system and improve mental health. While it is important to consume a healthy diet rich in fiber and probiotics to support a healthy microbiome, it is equally important to avoid certain foods and behaviors that can harm our gut bacteria. A high intake of processed foods, sugar, and saturated fats can disrupt the balance of our microbiome and promote the growth of harmful bacteria. The overuse of antibiotics can also have a detrimental effect on our gut bacteria. Antibiotics are designed to kill bacteria, both harmful and beneficial ones. While they may be necessary in certain situations, the overuse or misuse of antibiotics can lead to the destruction of our beneficial bacteria, causing an imbalance in our microbiome. It is crucial to use antibiotics judiciously and only when necessary. Understanding the science of the microbiome and its impact on our health is crucial for promoting optimal nutrition and overall well-being. The microbiome, particularly the gut microbiome, plays a vital role in our digestion, immune system, and overall health. Various factors, including diet, can influence the composition and function of our microbiome. Consuming a healthy diet rich in fiber and probiotics, while avoiding harmful foods and behaviors, can support the growth of beneficial bacteria and maintain a diverse and stable microbiome. By nourishing our gut bacteria, we can improve our overall health and well-being, promoting holistic wellness.

III. THE IMPACT OF THE MICROBIOME ON HUMAN HEALTH

The impact of the microbiome on human health is a topic of growing interest and research. The microbiome refers to the collection of microorganisms, including bacteria, viruses, fungi, and other microbes, that inhabit the human body. These microbes play a crucial role in maintaining our health by performing various functions such as aiding in digestion, synthesizing vitamins, and training our immune system. The delicate balance of the microbiome can be easily disrupted by factors such as poor diet, stress, antibiotics, and other environmental influences. This disruption, known as dysbiosis, has been linked to a wide range of health conditions, including obesity, diabetes, autoimmune diseases, and mental health disorders. One of the key areas in which the microbiome exerts its influence is on our immune system. The gut microbiome, in particular, plays a vital role in training our immune system to distinguish between harmless and harmful pathogens. It does this by interacting directly with immune cells and influencing their development and function. When the gut microbiome is in balance, it helps to prevent overactivation of the immune system and the development of chronic inflammation. When the microbiome is disrupted, the immune system can become dysregulated, leading to increased inflammation and the development of autoimmune diseases such as Crohn's disease and rheumatoid arthritis.

The microbiome also plays a crucial role in digestion and nutrient absorption. The diverse community of bacteria in our gut helps to break down complex carbohydrates and fiber that are otherwise indigestible by our own enzymes. These bacteria ferment these fibers and produce short-chain fatty acids, which serve as an important energy source for the cells lining our gut. In addition, the microbiome helps to produce enzymes that aid in the digestion and absorption of nutrients such as vitamins and minerals. Thus, a healthy microbiome is essential for proper nutrient absorption and overall digestion.

Recent studies have shown that the microbiome may also have an impact on our mental health. The gut-brain axis, a bidirectional communication system between our gut and our brain, allows the microbiome to influence our mood, behavior, and cognitive function. It is believed that the microbiome produces various metabolites, such as neurotransmitters and short-chain fatty acids, which can influence our brain chemistry and function. Dysbiosis of the microbiome has been linked to mental health disorders such as depression, anxiety, and even neurodegenerative diseases such as Alzheimer's and Parkinson's. Understanding this gut-brain connection is crucial for developing new therapies for mental health disorders that target the microbiome. Given the significant impact of the microbiome on human health, it is essential to consider how our diet and lifestyle choices can influence its composition and function. A diet rich in plant-based foods, such as fruits, vegetables, whole grains, and legumes, has been shown to promote a diverse and healthy microbiome. These foods are high in fiber, which acts as a prebiotic, providing nourishment for the beneficial bacteria in our gut. A diet high in processed foods, added sugars, and saturated fats has been shown to disrupt the microbiome and promote the growth of harmful bacteria.

In addition to diet, other lifestyle factors such as stress and antibiotic use can also impact the microbiome. Chronic stress has been shown to alter the composition of the gut microbiome and increase the risk of dysbiosis. Antibiotics, while necessary for treating bacterial infections, can also disrupt the balance of the microbiome by killing off beneficial bacteria along with the harmful ones. It is important to be mindful of these factors and take steps to promote a healthy microbiome through stress management techniques, judicious use of antibiotics, and the adoption of a balanced and varied diet.

The impact of the microbiome on human health is significant and wide-ranging. The microbiome plays a crucial role in immune function, digestion, nutrient absorption, and even mental health. Dysbiosis of the microbiome has been linked to a variety of health conditions, highlighting the importance of maintaining a healthy and diverse microbiome. To achieve this, it is essential to adopt a balanced and varied diet, manage stress levels, and be mindful of the use of antibiotics. By understanding and harnessing the power of the microbiome, we can optimize our health and well-being for a more holistic approach to nutrition.

THE LINK BETWEEN A HEALTHY MICROBIOME AND OVERALL WELLNESS

The link between a healthy microbiome and overall wellness extends beyond just physical health. Research has shown that the gut microbiome, in particular, plays a significant role in mental well-being as well. The gut-brain axis is a bidirectional communication pathway between the gut and the brain, in which the microbiome acts as an intermediary. It is now well-established that alterations in the gut microbiota can lead to changes in brain function and behavior.

One way in which the gut microbiome influences mental health is through the production of neurotransmitters. Neurotransmitters are chemicals that transmit signals between nerve cells in the brain, and they play a crucial role in regulating mood, cognition, and behavior. It is estimated that 90% of serotonin, a neurotransmitter associated with feelings of happiness and well-being, is produced in the gut. This means that an imbalance in the gut microbiome can affect serotonin production, leading to mood disorders such as depression and anxiety.

The gut microbiome also produces other neurotransmitters, such as gamma-aminobutyric acid (GABA) and dopamine, which have been shown to impact anxiety and reward pathways in the brain, respectively. In this way, the composition of the gut microbiota can influence mental health by modulating neurotransmitter production. In addition to neurotransmitters, the gut microbiome also produces and responds to other molecules that have an impact on brain function. For example, certain species of gut bacteria produce short-chain fatty acids (SCFAs) as a byproduct of fermenting dietary fibers. SCFAs, such as butyrate, have been shown to have anti-inflammatory and neuroprotective effects in the brain. They can enhance the integrity of the blood-brain barrier, reduce neuroinflammation, and promote the growth of new neurons. Conversely, dysbiosis, or an imbalance in the gut microbiota, has been associated with increased permeability of the blood-brain barrier and neuroinflammation, which are implicated in various neurological disorders, including Alzheimer's disease and multiple sclerosis.

The gut microbiome can also influence the immune system, which has implications for mental health. The gut is home to the largest population of immune cells in the body, and the microbiome plays a crucial role in immune system development and regulation. Studies have shown that alterations in the gut microbiome can lead to dysregulation of the immune system, contributing to chronic inflammation, which has been linked to depression and other mood disorders. In addition to mental health, a healthy microbiome is also essential for maintaining a healthy weight. A growing body of evidence suggests that the composition of the gut microbiota plays a role in energy metabolism and the regulation of appetite. Studies in mice have demonstrated that transplanting the gut microbiota from lean individuals into germ-free mice can lead to weight loss, while transplanting the microbiota from obese individuals can lead to weight gain. These findings suggest that an imbalance in the gut microbiome, characterized by a reduction in beneficial bacteria and an overgrowth of harmful bacteria, can contribute to obesity and metabolic disorders. The gut microbiome can influence the metabolism of carbohydrates and fats, as well as the production of hormones that regulate appetite and satiety. For example, certain species of gut bacteria can break down dietary fibers into SCFAs, which can modulate the production of hormones such as glucagon-like peptide 1 (GLP-1) and peptide YY (PYY), both of which promote feelings of fullness and reduce food intake.

The link between a healthy microbiome and overall wellness is multifaceted. In addition to its crucial role in digestion and nutrient absorption, the gut microbiome plays a significant role in mental health, immune system function, and weight regulation. Optimizing our nutrition to support a healthy microbiome is essential for achieving holistic wellness. By consuming a diverse diet rich in fruits, vegetables, whole grains, and fermented foods, we can promote the growth of beneficial gut bacteria and maintain a healthy microbiome. Adopting healthy lifestyle habits, such as regular physical activity and stress management, can also contribute to a thriving microbiome and overall well-being.

AN IMBALANCED MICROBIOME CAN LEAD TO VARIOUS HEALTH ISSUES

An imbalanced microbiome, also known as dysbiosis, has been linked to a wide range of health issues. One of the most well-known conditions associated with dysbiosis is irritable bowel syndrome (IBS). Research has shown that individuals with IBS often have an altered gut microbiota composition, characterized by a decrease in beneficial bacteria and an increase in pathogenic bacteria. This imbalance in the gut microbiome can lead to symptoms such as abdominal pain, bloating, and altered bowel habits. Dysbiosis has also been implicated in the development of inflammatory bowel diseases (IBD), including Crohn's disease and ulcerative colitis. In these conditions, an imbalanced microbiome can trigger chronic inflammation in the gut, leading to damage of the intestinal lining and various symptoms such as diarrhea, rectal bleeding, and weight loss.

Aside from gut-related disorders, dysbiosis has also been associated with metabolic disorders. One such disorder is obesity, which has reached epidemic proportions in many parts of the world. Recent studies have shown that individuals with obesity have a different gut microbial profile compared to those with a normal weight. Specifically, they tend to have a lower abundance of beneficial bacteria, such as Bacteroidetes, and a higher abundance of harmful bacteria, such as Firmicutes. This altered microbiome composition has been linked to increased extraction of energy from the diet and enhanced storage of fat, leading to weight gain and obesity. Interestingly, the gut microbiota composition can also influence our food preferences and cravings. Certain bacteria have been found to release compounds that stimulate the reward centers of the brain, increasing the desire for unhealthy, calorie-dense foods. This vicious cycle of imbalanced microbiota and weight gain creates a significant barrier for individuals trying to achieve a healthy weight. In addition to metabolic disorders, an imbalanced microbiome has also been implicated in mental health conditions. Studies have revealed a strong connection between the gut and the brain, known as the gut-brain axis. Dysbiosis of the gut microbiota has been associated with various mental health disorders, including anxiety and depression. For example, individuals with depression often exhibit differences in their gut microbiota composition, with a decrease in beneficial bacteria such as Bifidobacterium and Lactobacillus. This altered microbiome can lead to increased production of pro-inflammatory molecules and decreased production of neurotransmitters such as serotonin, which plays a vital role in mood regulation. Recent research has found a link between the gut microbiota and autism spectrum disorder (ASD). Children with ASD have been shown to have a different gut microbial profile compared to their neurotypical counterparts, with lower diversity and altered composition. This dysbiosis may contribute to the symptoms observed in ASD, such as social and communication difficulties, repetitive behaviors, and sensory sensitivities. An imbalanced microbiome has been associated with various autoimmune diseases, such as rheumatoid arthritis and multiple sclerosis. These conditions arise when the immune system mistakenly attacks the body's own tissues. The gut microbiota plays a crucial role in maintaining the balance between immune activation and tolerance.

Dysbiosis can disrupt this delicate balance, leading to an overactive immune response and chronic inflammation. In rheumatoid arthritis, for instance, studies have shown that certain bacteria in the gut can induce the production of antibodies that attack the joints. This immune response leads to joint inflammation, pain, and eventually, joint damage. Similarly, in multiple sclerosis, dysbiosis has been associated with a breakdown of the blood-brain barrier, allowing immune cells to enter the central nervous system and attack the protective covering of nerve fibers. These findings highlight the importance of a balanced microbiome in preventing autoimmune diseases and maintaining immune homeostasis. An imbalanced microbiome can have profound effects on our health and well-being. It can contribute to the development of various health issues, including gastrointestinal disorders, metabolic disorders, mental health conditions, and autoimmune diseases. Understanding the role of the microbiome in these diseases is crucial for developing targeted interventions and therapies. Through proper nutrition and lifestyle modifications, we can support a diverse and balanced microbiome, which is essential for maintaining our overall health and well-being. By optimizing our nutrition and taking steps to promote a healthy microbiome, we can empower ourselves to live a life of holistic wellness.

EXAMPLES OF SPECIFIC DISEASES OR CONDITIONS THAT ARE INFLUENCED BY THE MICROBIOME

The microbiome plays a crucial role in various diseases and conditions, further emphasizing its importance in our overall health. One such example is inflammatory bowel disease (IBD). IBD encompasses conditions like Crohn's disease and ulcerative colitis, which are characterized by chronic inflammation in the digestive tract. Studies have shown that the gut microbiota of individuals with IBD is altered, with reduced microbial diversity and an increase in potentially harmful bacteria. This dysbiosis can contribute to the inflammation observed in these individuals. Interestingly, the gut microbiota composition can also determine the response to certain therapies. For instance, individuals with certain bacterial species are more likely to respond to anti-TNF treatment, highlighting the potential to personalize treatments based on an individual's microbiome profile.

Another disease influenced by the microbiome is obesity. Obesity has become a global epidemic, and recent research suggests that alterations in the gut microbiome may contribute to this condition. Studies on both human and animal models have shown that the gut microbiota of obese individuals differs from that of lean individuals. The gut microbiota of obese individuals is characterized by a lower abundance of beneficial bacteria and an increase in bacteria associated with obesity-related metabolic conditions. Studies have demonstrated that transferring fecal matter from obese individuals to germ-free mice can induce weight gain, further emphasizing the role of the microbiome in obesity. This suggests that targeting the gut microbiota may hold promise in the management and prevention of obesity. The microbiome has been implicated in various mental health conditions, including depression and anxiety. The gut-brain axis, a bidirectional communication pathway between the gut and the central nervous system, is thought to be involved in this relationship. Studies have shown that alterations in the gut microbiota can influence brain function and behavior. For example, germ-free mice exhibit altered levels of neurotransmitters and increased anxiety-like behavior. In humans, research has shown that individuals with depression have altered gut microbiota composition, with lower levels of beneficial bacteria. Preliminary studies have shown that certain probiotics can improve symptoms of depression and anxiety. These findings suggest that targeting the gut microbiome may have potential therapeutic implications for mental health disorders.

In addition to diseases, the microbiome also influences the development of allergies and autoimmune conditions. Allergies involve an inappropriate immune response to harmless substances, while autoimmune conditions occur when the immune system attacks the body's own tissues. The gut microbiota plays a crucial role in the development and function of the immune system, and alterations in the microbiome composition can disrupt immune homeostasis. For instance, studies have shown that early exposure to a diverse range of microorganisms, including those found in the gut, can reduce the risk of developing allergies later in life. Conversely, an imbalance in the gut microbiota has been implicated in the development of autoimmune conditions such as rheumatoid arthritis and multiple sclerosis. These observations highlight the potential of modulating the gut microbiota to prevent and treat allergies and autoimmune conditions. The examples discussed above demonstrate the influence of the microbiome on various diseases and conditions. Understanding the intricate relationship between our bodies and the microorganisms within them is crucial for improving our health. The emerging field of microbiome research has opened new avenues for personalized medicine, where treatments can be tailored based on an individual's microbiome profile. Research on the microbiome has highlighted the importance of a holistic approach to health, where nutrition plays a key role in shaping our microbiome and overall well-being. As we continue to unravel the complexities of the microbiome, it is clear that optimizing nutrition and targeting the microbiome can pave the way for improved health outcomes and a better quality of life.

The field of microbiome research has emerged as a revolutionary area of study that has the potential to unlock new insights into human health and wellness. The microbiome refers to the vast community of microorganisms that reside within and on the human body. This community includes bacteria, viruses, fungi, and other microbes, and it is estimated that there are trillions of these organisms living within us. These microorganisms play a crucial role in maintaining our overall health and well-being by contributing to various physiological processes and interacting with our immune system. Researchers have begun to unravel the complex interactions between the microbiome and human health, and their findings have led to a paradigm shift in our understanding of optimal nutrition.

One of the key insights from microbiome research is that our diet has a significant impact on the composition and diversity of our microbiota. It has been found that certain dietary patterns can promote the growth of beneficial microorganisms, while others can disrupt the delicate balance of the microbiome and contribute to disease development. For example, a diet high in processed foods and added sugars has been shown to promote the growth of harmful bacteria in the gut, such as Firmicutes, while a diet rich in fiber and plant-based foods can enhance the abundance of beneficial bacteria, such as Bacteroidetes. These findings highlight the importance of adopting a diet that is aligned with our evolutionary history and supports the growth of a diverse and balanced microbiota. Another important aspect of nutrition that has been linked to microbial health is the concept of prebiotics and probiotics. Prebiotics are a type of dietary fiber that cannot be broken down by our digestive enzymes, but instead, serve as a fuel source for beneficial bacteria in the gut. By consuming prebiotic-rich foods, such as asparagus, onions, and bananas, we can selectively promote the growth of beneficial bacteria and improve the overall health of our microbiome. Probiotics, on the other hand, are live microorganisms that, when consumed in adequate amounts, confer a health benefit on the host. These can be found in fermented foods such as yogurt, sauerkraut, and kimchi. By incorporating prebiotics and probiotics into our diet, we can promote the growth of beneficial bacteria and create an environment that is conducive to optimal health. In addition to diet, there are other lifestyle factors that can influence the composition and diversity of our microbiome. For instance, exercise has been shown to have a positive impact on the microbiota, with studies demonstrating that physically active individuals have a more diverse and beneficial microbiome compared to sedentary individuals. Stress levels have also been found to impact the microbiota, with chronic stress leading to alterations in the composition of the gut microbiome and an increased risk of various health conditions. Sleep deprivation has been shown to alter the gut microbiome in a way that is similar to an unhealthy diet, with a decrease in beneficial bacteria and an increase in harmful bacteria. These findings highlight the significance of adopting a holistic approach to health and wellness, where nutrition, exercise, stress management, and sleep are all considered. Understanding the intricate relationship between the microbiome and human health has far-reaching implications for various areas of medicine. For example, researchers are exploring the potential of manipulating the microbiome to treat and prevent a range of conditions, including obesity, Type 2 diabetes, inflammatory bowel disease, and even mental health disorders such as depression and anxiety. By understanding the specific microbial signatures associated with these conditions, scientists can develop targeted interventions, such as personalized diets and probiotic therapies, to restore microbial balance and improve patient outcomes.

The microbiome is a fascinating area of research that has the potential to revolutionize our understanding of human health and wellness. Through the study of the microbiome, we have discovered the profound impact that diet and lifestyle factors have on our microbial health and overall well-being. By adopting a diet rich in prebiotic and probiotic foods, engaging in regular exercise, managing stress levels, and prioritizing sleep, we can create an environment that promotes the growth of beneficial bacteria and supports optimal health. The emerging field of microbiome therapeutics holds promise for the development of targeted interventions to treat and prevent a range of diseases. With continued research and exploration, we can harness the power of the microbiome to improve our health and well-being in a holistic and sustainable way.

IV. OPTIMAL NUTRITION FOR A HEALTHY MICROBIOME

Maintaining a healthy microbiome is essential for overall wellness, and one crucial factor in achieving this balance is through optimal nutrition. The foods we consume have a significant impact on the composition and diversity of our microbiomes, ultimately affecting various aspects of our health. Research has shown that a diet rich in fiber, prebiotics, and fermented foods is beneficial for nurturing a healthy microbiome. Fiber serves as a vital fuel source for the gut bacteria, allowing them to thrive and perform their functions effectively. Prebiotics, such as inulin and resistant starch, act as nourishment for the beneficial bacteria in our guts, promoting their growth and activity. These substances can be found abundantly in fruits, vegetables, whole grains, and legumes, emphasizing the importance of incorporating these foods into our diets. Fermented foods, such as yogurt, sauerkraut, and kimchi, are excellent sources of probiotics. Probiotics are beneficial bacteria that can colonize our intestines and contribute to a healthy microbiome. Consuming these foods can help replenish and diversify the microbial communities in our gut, enhancing its overall balance. In addition to their direct impact on the microbiome, fermented foods also provide essential nutrients and can improve our digestion. Including a variety of fermented foods in our diet can help support the growth of beneficial bacteria and maintain a thriving microbiome.

In contrast, a diet lacking in fiber and high in unhealthy fats, added sugars, and processed foods can have detrimental effects on the microbiome. Studies have shown that a Western-style diet, characterized by a high consumption of refined grains, sugary beverages, red meat, and processed snacks, is associated with a reduced diversity of gut bacteria and an imbalance in microbial composition. This imbalance, known as dysbiosis, has been linked to various health issues, including obesity, type 2 diabetes, and inflammatory bowel disease.

Understanding the specific nutrients that promote a healthy microbiome is crucial in optimizing our nutrition for holistic wellness. For example, the short-chain fatty acids (SCFAs) produced by gut bacteria during the fermentation of dietary fiber have been recognized as essential for maintaining a healthy gut environment. SCFAs, such as acetate, propionate, and butyrate, not only provide an energy source for colon cells but also possess anti-inflammatory properties. These molecules play a vital role in enhancing gut barrier function, reducing the risk of inflammation-related conditions, and supporting overall immune health.

Certain nutrients, such as polyphenols, have been shown to exert prebiotic-like effects, promoting the growth of beneficial bacteria in the gut. Polyphenols, found abundantly in fruits, vegetables, and teas, have been associated with increased microbial diversity and improved gut health. Their antioxidant and anti-inflammatory properties contribute to a healthy microbiome by reducing oxidative stress and modulating immune responses. In addition to incorporating specific nutrients for a healthy microbiome, it is essential to adopt a balanced, varied, and unprocessed diet. By focusing on whole foods rather than highly processed alternatives, we can ensure that we are providing our bodies with the necessary nutrients for optimal health. Whole foods, such as fruits, vegetables, whole grains, and lean proteins, contain a wide range of vitamins, minerals, and phytochemicals that have positive effects on our gut bacteria and overall well-being. Optimal nutrition plays a crucial role in maintaining a healthy microbiome, which is essential for our overall wellness. Consuming a diet rich in fiber, prebiotics, and fermented foods can nurture a flourishing and diverse microbial community in our guts. These foods provide essential nutrients for our gut bacteria, promoting their growth, activity, and overall balance. Conversely, a diet high in unhealthy fats, added sugars, and processed foods can disrupt the microbial composition and diversity, leading to dysbiosis and associated health issues. Understanding the specific nutrients that promote a healthy microbiome, such as fiber, prebiotics, SCFAs, and polyphenols, allows us to make informed choices about our dietary habits. By adopting a balanced, varied, and unprocessed diet, we can optimize our nutrition to support a thriving microbiome and improve our overall health and well-being.

THE CONCEPT OF OPTIMAL NUTRITION AND ITS IMPORTANCE FOR THE MICROBIOME

The concept of optimal nutrition is centered around providing the body with the necessary nutrients in the right quantities to maintain good health and prevent chronic diseases. When it comes to the microbiome, optimal nutrition refers to consuming a diverse and balanced diet that supports the growth and diversity of beneficial microbes in the gut. These beneficial microbes carry out essential functions that contribute to our overall well-being. One of the key reasons why optimal nutrition is important for the microbiome is its role in supporting a diverse community of beneficial microbes. The gut microbiome is comprised of trillions of microorganisms, including bacteria, viruses, fungi, and other microbes. This vast community functions as a complex ecosystem that interacts with the host's body and plays a critical role in various physiological processes.

Diet has a profound impact on the composition and activity of the gut microbiome. Certain dietary components, such as dietary fiber, serve as a source of energy for beneficial microbes in the gut. These microbes ferment dietary fiber to produce short-chain fatty acids (SCFAs), which serve as an energy source for the cells lining the gut and have anti-inflammatory effects. Inadequate intake of dietary fiber can lead to a reduction in the diversity and abundance of beneficial microbes, negatively impacting the overall health of the gut microbiome.

In addition to dietary fiber, other components of a healthy diet also play a crucial role in supporting a diverse and balanced gut microbiome. For example, consuming a variety of plant-based foods rich in polyphenols, such as fruits, vegetables, nuts, and whole grains, helps promote the growth of beneficial microbes. Polyphenols are bioactive compounds that have been shown to have antimicrobial, anti-inflammatory, and antioxidant properties. They can modulate the composition of the gut microbiota and promote the growth of beneficial bacteria, such as lactobacillus and bifidobacteria, while inhibiting the growth of harmful bacteria. The consumption of adequate amounts of protein is also important for maintaining a healthy gut microbiome. Protein serves as a source of essential amino acids that are necessary for the growth and proliferation of beneficial microbes. Certain amino acids, such as tryptophan, can be metabolized by gut bacteria into neurotransmitters, such as serotonin, which regulates mood and mental health.

Optimal nutrition is not just about consuming the right nutrients, but also about avoiding certain dietary factors that can negatively impact the gut microbiome. For instance, excessive consumption of highly processed foods, saturated fats, and added sugars has been associated with an imbalance in the gut microbiota, known as dysbiosis. Dysbiosis is characterized by a reduction in the abundance of beneficial microbes and an overgrowth of harmful bacteria, which can lead to various health problems, such as obesity, metabolic disorders, and inflammatory bowel diseases. Optimal nutrition is vital for the microbiome as it supports the growth and diversity of beneficial microbes in the gut. A diverse and balanced diet, rich in dietary fiber, polyphenols, and protein, promotes the growth of beneficial bacteria and helps maintain a healthy gut microbiome. A diet high in processed foods, saturated fats, and added sugars can disrupt the balance of the gut microbiota, leading to dysbiosis and an increased risk of chronic diseases. Understanding the concept of optimal nutrition and its importance for the microbiome is crucial for improving our overall health and well-being.

THE KEY NUTRIENTS AND DIETARY COMPONENTS THAT PROMOTE A HEALTHY MICROBIOME

The key nutrients and dietary components that promote a healthy microbiome play a vital role in maintaining our overall health and well-being. One such component is fiber, which is found in abundance in fruits, vegetables, and whole grains. Fiber acts as a prebiotic, providing fuel for the beneficial bacteria in our gut. These bacteria ferment fiber and produce short-chain fatty acids, such as butyrate, which have been shown to have numerous health benefits. Butyrate, for example, has anti-inflammatory properties and helps to maintain the integrity of the gut barrier. In addition to fiber, polyphenols also have a positive impact on the microbiome. Polyphenols are found in foods such as berries, dark chocolate, and green tea. They act as antioxidants, protecting our cells from damage caused by free radicals. Recent research has shown that polyphenols also have an anti-inflammatory effect and can promote the growth of beneficial bacteria in the gut. Another key nutrient for a healthy microbiome is omega-3 fatty acids. These essential fats are found in fatty fish, walnuts, and flaxseeds. Omega-3 fatty acids have been shown to reduce inflammation in the body and support the growth of beneficial bacteria in the gut. They have also been linked to improvements in mood and mental health. Vitamin D, another important nutrient for a healthy microbiome, is synthesized in the skin when exposed to sunlight. Vitamin D plays a crucial role in immune function and has been shown to modulate the composition of the gut microbiome. Low levels of vitamin D have been associated with dysbiosis, an imbalance of bacteria in the gut that can lead to various health issues. Probiotics, which are live bacteria or yeasts that confer a health benefit when consumed, also play a key role in maintaining a healthy microbiome. Probiotics can be found in fermented foods such as yogurt, sauerkraut, and kefir. These probiotics help to restore the balance of bacteria in the gut and promote a healthy digestive system. It is also important to note that not all fats are detrimental to the microbiome. In fact, some fats are essential for its optimal function. For example, medium-chain triglycerides (MCTs), found in coconut oil, are easily digested and absorbed by the body. They can provide a readily available source of energy for the gut bacteria and help to maintain a healthy microbiome. In contrast, a diet high in saturated and trans fats can promote the growth of harmful bacteria in the gut and disrupt the balance of the microbiome. It is important to consider the role of artificial sweeteners in the microbiome. These non-nutritive sweeteners, such as aspartame and sucralose, are commonly used as sugar substitutes in many processed foods and beverages. Studies have shown that artificial sweeteners can negatively impact the composition of the gut microbiome. These sweeteners can alter the balance of bacteria in the gut, leading to metabolic dysfunction and an increased risk of obesity and other chronic diseases. The key nutrients and dietary components that promote a healthy microbiome are essential for maintaining our overall health and well-being. Fiber, polyphenols, omega-3 fatty acids, vitamin D, and probiotics all play crucial roles in supporting the growth of beneficial bacteria and maintaining a balanced microbiome. Consuming high amounts of saturated and trans fats and artificial sweeteners can disrupt

the microbiome and lead to various health issues. By understanding the importance of these nutrients and making conscious choices about the foods we consume, we can optimize
our gut health and improve our overall wellness.

THE IMPORTANCE OF A DIVERSE AND BALANCED DIET FOR MICROBIOME HEALTH

The microbiome, consisting of trillions of microorganisms that inhabit our bodies, has emerged as a topic of great interest due to its profound effects on human health. Researchers have discovered that the diversity and composition of our gut microbiota can influence various aspects of our well-being, including immune function, metabolism, and mental health. One crucial factor that determines the health of our microbiome is the food we consume. A diverse and balanced diet is vital for maintaining a healthy microbiome because it ensures the presence of a wide array of beneficial microorganisms while limiting the growth of harmful bacteria. A diverse diet rich in different types of fiber is essential for the health and diversity of our microbiome. Fiber, found in fruits, vegetables, whole grains, and legumes, serves as a valuable food source for the bacteria residing in our gut. Not all fiber is created equal. Different types of fiber, such as soluble and insoluble fiber, are fermented by different groups of bacteria, leading to the production of various beneficial metabolites. This fermentation process produces short-chain fatty acids (SCFAs), such as butyrate, acetate, and propionate, which provide energy to the cells lining our intestines and exert anti-inflammatory effects. A diverse diet helps maintain the balance between beneficial and harmful bacteria in the gut. The presence of a wide range of microorganisms ensures that no single species dominates, preventing overgrowth of certain bacteria that could be detrimental to our health. For instance, a lack of dietary diversity has been associated with a decrease in microbial richness and an increase in the abundance of harmful bacteria, such as Clostridium difficile. This imbalance, known as dysbiosis, has been linked to various conditions, including inflammatory bowel disease, irritable bowel syndrome, and obesity. In addition to promoting microbial diversity, a balanced diet that contains the right proportions of macronutrients is crucial for microbiome health. It is well-known that excessive consumption of certain macronutrients, such as fats and simple sugars, can disrupt the balance of gut bacteria and promote the growth of harmful species. A high-fat diet, for example, has been shown to increase the abundance of bacteria associated with inflammation and metabolic disorders, such as Firmicutes. A diet rich in plant-based foods, low in added sugars, and moderate in healthy fats, such as those found in nuts, olive oil, and fatty fish, has been associated with a more favorable microbiome composition and improved metabolic health. The importance of a diverse and balanced diet extends beyond the gut microbiome. Recent studies have revealed the existence of a gut-brain axis, a bidirectional communication pathway between the gut and the brain, through which the microbiome can influence brain function and behavior. A growing body of evidence suggests that an imbalance in the microbial community can contribute to the development of mental health disorders such as anxiety and depression. Interestingly, the Mediterranean diet, characterized by its abundance of plant-based foods, fish, and healthy fats, has been associated with a decreased risk of depression. This diet, rich in fiber and prebiotics, promotes the growth of beneficial bacteria that produce serotonin, a neurotransmitter involved in mood regulation.

Maintaining a diverse and balanced diet is essential for nurturing a healthy microbiome, with wide-ranging implications for our overall health and well-being. A diverse diet rich in fiber promotes microbial diversity, enables the production of beneficial metabolites, and helps maintain the balance between beneficial and harmful bacteria in the gut. A balanced diet that contains the right proportions of macronutrients ensures the stability of the gut microbiota and supports metabolic health. The gut microbiome's influence on mental health highlights the importance of dietary choices in promoting holistic wellness. By embracing a diverse and balanced diet, we can optimize our microbiome and take a significant step towards achieving optimal health. One of the primary factors that influence the health of our microbiome is the food we consume. The foods we eat provide essential nutrients for the growth and maintenance of the diverse microbial communities within our bodies. It is widely accepted that a balanced and diverse diet is key to achieving optimal nutrition and promoting overall health.

Dietary fibers are particularly essential for the well-being of our microbiome. These fibers are indigestible by our own enzymes, but they serve as an important fuel source for the bacteria residing in our gut. When we consume dietary fibers, they travel to the colon, where they are fermented by our gut bacteria. As a result of this fermentation process, various beneficial compounds are produced, such as short-chain fatty acids (SCFAs).

SCFAs are known to have numerous health benefits. They serve as an energy source for the cells lining our colon, help regulate our immune system, and play a crucial role in maintaining a healthy gut barrier. SCFAs have been linked to reduced inflammation, improved insulin sensitivity, and a lower risk of chronic diseases, such as obesity, type 2 diabetes, and cardiovascular disease. Including an adequate amount of dietary fibers in our diet is vital for nurturing a healthy microbiome and promoting overall wellness. Another aspect of optimal nutrition that significantly impacts our microbiome is the diversity of our diet. Consuming a wide variety of foods ensures that we are exposed to different types of nutrients and compounds that can support the growth of different beneficial bacteria within our gut. Studies have shown that individuals with a more diverse diet tend to have a more diverse and resilient microbiome. A diet lacking in variety may lead to a reduction in microbial diversity, which has been associated with various health problems, including obesity and gastrointestinal disorders. In addition to dietary fibers and diversity, the balance between different types of nutrients is also crucial for the health of our microbiome. For example, excessive consumption of saturated fats and added sugars has been shown to promote the growth of harmful bacteria and negatively impact the diversity of our gut microbiota. Diets rich in fruits, vegetables, whole grains, and lean proteins tend to promote the growth of beneficial bacteria and support a healthy microbiome. The impact of certain dietary patterns on our microbiome and overall health has been extensively studied. For instance, the Mediterranean diet, which is rich in fruits, vegetables, whole grains, lean proteins, and healthy fats, has been associated with a more diverse and beneficial gut microbiome. This dietary pattern has also been linked to a lower risk of chronic diseases, such as heart disease and certain types of cancer. It is important to acknowledge that the effect of diet on the microbiome varies among individuals. Factors such as genetics, age, gender, and lifestyle can influence how our microbiome responds to different types of foods. It is crucial to take a personalized approach to nutrition and consider individual differences when designing dietary recommendations for optimal microbiome health. Optimal nutrition plays a significant role in supporting a healthy microbiome and promoting overall wellness. Including a variety of dietary fibers in our diet, consuming a diverse range of foods, and maintaining a balanced nutrient intake are essential for nurturing a beneficial and resilient gut microbiota. By understanding the science behind the microbiome and its interactions with our diet, we can make informed choices about the foods we consume and proactively improve our health and well-being.

V. THE ROLE OF PROBIOTICS AND PREBIOTICS IN OPTIMAL NUTRITION

Probiotics and prebiotics play a crucial role in achieving optimal nutrition and holistic wellness. Probiotics, which are live bacteria that are beneficial to the host, can enhance our gut health by maintaining the balance of our microbiome. Their ability to improve digestion and absorption of nutrients, strengthen the immune system, and reduce inflammation makes them a valuable addition to our diet. Through their production of short-chain fatty acids and other metabolites, they can modulate host metabolism, metabolism, and gene expression, promoting overall health and preventing chronic diseases. Probiotics have been shown to provide relief from common digestive disorders such as irritable bowel syndrome (IBS) and inflammatory bowel disease (IBD). These findings highlight the potential of probiotics as therapeutic agents, providing a natural and side effect-free alternative to conventional medication.

Similarly, prebiotics also have a significant impact on our microbiome and overall well-being. Prebiotics are non-digestible fibers that serve as food for the beneficial bacteria in our gut, stimulating their growth and activity. As a result, prebiotics can contribute to a more diverse and robust microbiome, which is associated with improved health outcomes. They can also enhance the production of short-chain fatty acids, which play a crucial role in maintaining gut integrity and function. By nourishing our gut bacteria, prebiotics can promote optimal digestion and absorption of nutrients, reduce the risk of certain diseases, and improve immune function.

Incorporating probiotics and prebiotics into our diet can be achieved through various food sources. Fermented foods like yogurt, kefir, sauerkraut, and kimchi are rich in live and active cultures, making them excellent sources of probiotics. These traditional foods have been consumed for centuries and are known for their health benefits. In addition, there are now many probiotic supplements available in the market, which can be useful for individuals with specific health concerns or those who have difficulty obtaining probiotics from their diet alone.

Prebiotics, on the other hand, are found in a wide range of plant-based foods, especially those that are rich in dietary fiber. Fruits, vegetables, whole grains, and legumes are all excellent sources of prebiotic fibers. By including a variety of these foods in our daily diet, we can nourish our gut bacteria and promote a healthy microbiome. It is important to note that probiotics and prebiotics work synergistically, and consuming them together can have an even greater impact on our gut health and overall well-being. While probiotics and prebiotics are generally safe for consumption, it is essential to consider individual differences and potential interactions, especially for those with underlying health conditions or compromised immune systems. Consultation with a healthcare professional is recommended before starting any probiotic or prebiotic supplementation, particularly for individuals with specific health concerns or those taking medications that may be affected by these interventions.

The role of probiotics and prebiotics in optimal nutrition cannot be overstated. They are fundamental in nurturing a healthy microbiome, which has far-reaching effects on our overall health and well-being. From improving digestion and nutrient absorption to boosting immune function and preventing chronic diseases, probiotics and prebiotics have proven their worth in the realm of nutritional science. Incorporating probiotics and prebiotics into our diet through fermented foods and plant-based sources of fiber is a practical and accessible way to support our microbiome. It is crucial to consider individual variations and potential interactions and to seek professional advice before starting any supplementation. By understanding and harnessing the power of probiotics and prebiotics, we can pave the way towards optimal nutrition and holistic wellness.

THE DIFFERENCE BETWEEN PROBIOTICS AND PREBIOTICS

Probiotics and prebiotics are two terms that are often used interchangeably, but they actually refer to different components of our digestive system. Probiotics are living microorganisms, such as bacteria or yeast, that are beneficial to our health when consumed in adequate amounts. These organisms help maintain a balanced gut microbiome by inhibiting the growth of harmful bacteria and promoting the growth of beneficial bacteria. They can be found naturally in certain foods, such as yogurt, sauerkraut, and kimchi, or can be taken as supplements. Prebiotics, on the other hand, are non-digestible fiber compounds that serve as food for probiotics. They cannot be broken down by our digestive enzymes, so they reach the colon largely intact, where they can be fermented by the gut bacteria. This fermentation process produces short-chain fatty acids, which provide energy to the cells in our colon and also have anti-inflammatory properties. Some examples of prebiotic-rich foods include whole grains, legumes, onions, garlic, and artichokes. While probiotics and prebiotics are different components, they work synergistically to promote a healthy gut microbiome and overall well-being. One of the key differences between probiotics and prebiotics lies in their composition and function. Probiotics are living microorganisms that are introduced into the body either through natural food sources or supplements. Once ingested, these microorganisms can colonize the gut and have various beneficial effects on our health. For example, some strains of bacteria in probiotics can help enhance our immune system, improve digestion, and even reduce the risk of certain diseases. They can also contribute to the production of vitamins, such as vitamin K and some B vitamins, which are essential for our overall health. In contrast, prebiotics are non-living components and consist of dietary fiber that cannot be digested by our own enzymes. Instead, they serve as fuel for beneficial bacteria in the gut. By providing these bacteria with the nutrients they need to thrive, prebiotics help maintain a diverse and balanced microbiome, which is crucial for our overall health and well-being.

Another important difference between probiotics and prebiotics is their source. Probiotics can be naturally found in certain foods or can be consumed in the form of supplements. There are many different strains of bacteria and yeast used as probiotics, each with their own specific benefits. For example, Lactobacillus and Bifidobacterium are two common genera of bacteria found in probiotic supplements that have been extensively studied for their health benefits. Prebiotics are mainly obtained through dietary sources. This means that by incorporating prebiotic-rich foods into our diet, we can support the growth of beneficial bacteria in our gut naturally. It is worth noting that both probiotics and prebiotics can be beneficial for our health, but they work through different mechanisms and have distinct roles in maintaining a healthy gut microbiome.

While probiotics and prebiotics have their own unique roles, they also complement each other in promoting a healthy gut microbiome. Probiotics help introduce beneficial microorganisms into the gut, while prebiotics serve as their food source, allowing them to thrive and exert their positive effects.

This synergistic relationship between probiotics and prebiotics is often referred to as synbiotics. Studies have shown that consuming both probiotics and prebiotics simultaneously can have a more significant impact on our gut microbiome compared to consuming them individually. This is because probiotics and prebiotics work together to create an environment that is conducive to the growth of beneficial bacteria, while inhibiting the growth of harmful bacteria. It is important to note that the effectiveness of probiotics and prebiotics can vary depending on the individual and the specific strains used, so it is essential to choose high-quality products and consult with a healthcare professional if needed. Probiotics and prebiotics are distinct components that play important roles in maintaining a healthy gut microbiome and overall well-being. Probiotics are living microorganisms that have various health benefits when consumed in adequate amounts, while prebiotics are non-digestible fibers that serve as food for these beneficial organisms. By working synergistically, probiotics and prebiotics contribute to a diverse and balanced microbiome, which is essential for our optimal nutrition and overall health. Incorporating probiotic-rich foods or supplements and prebiotic-rich foods into our diet can help support a healthy gut microbiome, enhance digestion, and potentially reduce the risk of certain diseases. Understanding the difference between probiotics and prebiotics and their roles in our digestive system can empower us to make informed decisions about our diet and lifestyle to promote optimal health.

PROBIOTICS AND PREBIOTICS CAN INFLUENCE THE MICROBIOME

Probiotics and prebiotics have gained significant attention in recent years due to their potential to shape and modulate the human microbiome, which is crucial for overall health and wellness. Probiotics are live microorganisms that, when consumed in adequate amounts, confer health benefits on the host.

These beneficial bacteria, such as Lactobacillus and Bifidobacterium species, can help restore the natural balance of the gut microbiota, which is essential for optimal digestion and immune function. These microorganisms can also produce metabolites that have anti-inflammatory and anti-cancer properties.

Studies have shown that probiotics have a diverse range of effects on the microbiome. For example, they can inhibit the growth of harmful pathogenic bacteria by producing antimicrobial substances, competing for nutrients, and lowering the pH in the intestines. They also enhance the integrity of the intestinal barrier, preventing the translocation of harmful bacteria and toxins into the bloodstream. Probiotics can modulate the immune system by increasing the production of anti-inflammatory cytokines and promoting the activity of immune cells. These effects can be particularly beneficial for individuals with gastrointestinal disorders, such as irritable bowel syndrome and inflammatory bowel disease. Prebiotics are non-digestible dietary fibers that selectively stimulate the growth and activity of beneficial bacteria in the gut. These compounds, including inulin, fructooligosaccharides, and resistant starch, serve as the preferred energy source for beneficial bacteria, allowing them to thrive and outcompete harmful microorganisms. Prebiotics can also stimulate the production of short-chain fatty acids (SCFAs), such as butyrate, which have numerous health benefits. SCFAs not only provide an energy source for the cells lining the colon but also exert anti-inflammatory effects, improve insulin sensitivity, and enhance satiety. Both probiotics and prebiotics can be consumed through dietary sources or as supplements. Fermented foods, such as yogurt, kefir, and sauerkraut, are rich sources of live probiotic bacteria. These foods undergo a fermentation process, in which beneficial bacteria convert sugars into lactic acid and other metabolites, creating an acidic environment that inhibits the growth of pathogens. It is important to note that not all fermented foods contain live probiotics, as some undergo pasteurization or other processes that kill the bacteria. In addition to dietary sources, probiotics are available in supplemental form, which allows for specific strains and dosages to be targeted. These supplements may be beneficial for individuals who have an imbalance in their gut microbiota or those who need a higher concentration of beneficial bacteria. It is worth noting that the effects of probiotics can vary depending on the strain, dosage, and individual characteristics, such as age, diet, and health status. It is recommended to consult with a healthcare professional before starting any probiotic supplementation. Similarly, prebiotics can be obtained from various dietary sources, including fruits, vegetables, whole grains, and legumes. Foods rich in dietary fiber, such as onions, garlic, bananas, and oats, are particularly good sources of prebiotics. Incorporating these foods into the diet can promote the growth of beneficial bacteria and improve overall gut health. It is important to gradually increase the intake of prebiotic-rich foods, as a sudden increase in fiber intake can cause digestive discomfort, such as bloating and gas. Probiotics and prebiotics play a crucial role in shaping and modulating the human microbiome, which has a significant impact on overall health and wellness. Probiotics can restore the balance of gut microbiota, inhibit the growth of harmful bacteria, and modulate the immune system. Prebiotics, on the other hand, selectively stimulate the growth of beneficial bacteria and promote the production of short-chain fatty acids, which have numerous health benefits. Both probiotics and prebiotics can be obtained through dietary sources or supplements and can be incorporated into a balanced and diverse diet for optimal gut health. Future research is needed to further understand the complex interactions between these microorganisms and their potential to improve human health.

THE FOOD SOURCES AND SUPPLEMENTS THAT PROVIDE PROBIOTICS AND PREBIOTICS

Probiotics and prebiotics have gained considerable attention in recent years due to their potential health benefits. Probiotics are live microorganisms that, when consumed in adequate amounts, confer a health benefit on the host. They are commonly found in fermented foods such as yogurt, kefir, sauerkraut, and kimchi. Yogurt is perhaps the most well-known source of probiotics and is widely consumed for its potential to support digestive health and boost the immune system. Kefir, a fermented milk drink, is another excellent probiotic source, rich in beneficial bacteria such as Lactobacillus and Bifidobacterium. These cultures aid in boosting gut health and can improve lactose digestion, particularly beneficial for individuals with lactose intolerance. Sauerkraut, a traditional fermented cabbage dish, contains lactic acid bacteria, which are known for their antimicrobial properties and ability to reduce inflammation in the gut. Kimchi, a Korean fermented vegetable dish, is a potent probiotic source and is rich in Lactobacillus and other beneficial bacteria. These traditional fermented foods have been consumed for centuries and are now being recognized for their role in promoting gut health and overall well-being. In addition to fermented foods, probiotics can also be obtained through dietary supplements. Probiotic supplements typically contain specific strains of bacteria that have been shown to confer health benefits. The strains commonly included in supplements include Lactobacillus acidophilus, Bifidobacterium lactis, and Saccharomyces boulardii. These supplements are a convenient way to increase probiotic intake, particularly for individuals who do not regularly consume fermented foods. While probiotics are live microorganisms, prebiotics are non-digestible fibers that serve as food for these beneficial bacteria. They help nourish the existing gut flora, supporting their growth and activity. Prebiotics can be found in certain plant-based foods, such as onions, garlic, leeks, asparagus, bananas, and chicory root. These foods are rich in various types of dietary fibers, including inulin and fructooligosaccharides, which are known to stimulate the growth of beneficial bacteria like Bifidobacterium and Lactobacillus. Whole grains, nuts, and seeds also contain prebiotic fibers that promote a healthy gut environment. There are prebiotic supplements available that can be taken to increase prebiotic intake. These supplements often contain fiber isolates, such as inulin or chicory root extract. They can be a convenient way to ensure an adequate intake of prebiotics, particularly for individuals who have dietary restrictions or difficulty incorporating prebiotic-rich foods into their diet. Both probiotics and prebiotics play a crucial role in maintaining a healthy gut microbiome, and research suggests that a balanced combination of the two can have synergistic effects on gut health. Consumption of probiotics and prebiotics has been associated with numerous health benefits, including improved digestion, enhanced nutrient absorption, strengthened immune function, and even mental health benefits. It is worth noting that the effects of probiotics and prebiotics can vary depending on the individual and the specific strains or types consumed. The composition of the gut microbiome is highly individualized, and factors such as genetics, diet, lifestyle, and medications can influence the response to probiotics and prebiotics. It is essential to consider these factors when incorporating probiotics and prebiotics into the diet.

Probiotics and prebiotics are important components of a healthy diet and have been shown to have numerous health benefits, particularly for gut health. Fermented foods such as yogurt, kefir, sauerkraut, and kimchi are excellent natural sources of probiotics. Dietary supplements can also provide a convenient way to increase probiotic intake. Prebiotics, on the other hand, can be obtained through various plant-based foods, including onions, garlic, leeks, asparagus, bananas, and chicory root. Prebiotic supplements can also be taken to ensure an adequate intake. Both probiotics and prebiotics work together to support a healthy gut microbiome and promote overall well-being. It is important to note that the effects of probiotics and prebiotics can vary among individuals, making it crucial to consider individual factors when incorporating them into the diet. By understanding the sources and benefits of probiotics and prebiotics, individuals can make informed choices to optimize their nutrition and improve their overall health. The microbiome, a community of microorganisms living in and on our bodies, is an emerging field of study that has revolutionized our understanding of human health. The microbiome consists of trillions of bacteria, viruses, and fungi that play a crucial role in maintaining our overall well-being. These microorganisms reside in various parts of our bodies, such as the gut, skin, and mouth, and actively interact with our cells, influencing our immune system, metabolism, and even our mental health. Recent research has shown that the microbiome is highly diverse, with each individual harboring a unique composition of microorganisms. The diversity of the microbiome is influenced by various factors, one of the most important being our diet.

Optimal nutrition is key to maintaining a healthy microbiome as the foods we eat directly influence the composition and functioning of our gut bacteria. The gut microbiome, in particular, is heavily influenced by our diet, as it directly interacts with the food that passes through our digestive system. Consuming a diet rich in fiber, whole grains, fruits, and vegetables promotes the growth of beneficial bacteria in the gut. These beneficial bacteria, known as probiotics, help in the digestion and absorption of food, produce essential vitamins, and strengthen our immune system. Fiber, in particular, plays a crucial role in nurturing a healthy gut microbiome. It is a type of carbohydrate that our bodies cannot digest, but it serves as food for beneficial gut bacteria. When we consume fiber-rich foods, such as whole grains, legumes, and fruits, our gut bacteria ferment the fiber and produce short-chain fatty acids (SCFAs). These SCFAs are not only a vital source of energy for the colon cells but also have anti-inflammatory properties and help maintain a healthy gut lining. Consequently, a diet lacking in fiber can lead to a depletion of beneficial gut bacteria, a decrease in SCFA production, and an increased risk of conditions like inflammation, diabetes, and obesity. In addition to fiber, prebiotics are another dietary component that plays a significant role in nurturing a healthy microbiome. Prebiotics are non-digestible compounds found in certain foods, such as onions, garlic, and asparagus, which selectively promote the growth of beneficial bacteria. By providing a nourishing environment for these bacteria, prebiotics help maintain a balanced and diverse gut microbiome. Including prebiotic-rich foods in our diet not only supports the growth of beneficial bacteria but also helps inhibit the growth of harmful bacteria, preventing infections and other gut disorders. A diet high in saturated fats and sugar promotes the growth of harmful bacteria in our gut, leading to an imbalance in the microbiome. These harmful bacteria produce toxic byproducts, such as lipopolysaccharides (LPS), which can trigger an inflammatory response in our bodies. Inflammation, especially chronic inflammation, is associated with numerous diseases, including cardiovascular diseases, type 2 diabetes, and certain types of cancer. Reducing the intake of processed foods, sugary beverages, and fatty meats is crucial for maintaining the health of our microbiome. The science of the microbiome has expanded beyond gut health and shed light on the link between the microbiome and mental health. The gut-brain axis, a bidirectional communication system between the gut microbiome and the brain, plays a crucial role in regulating our mood and behavior. It has been discovered that certain gut bacteria produce neurotransmitters, such as serotonin and dopamine, which are known to influence our mood and affect our mental well-being. The gut microbiome has been found to influence the stress response and even play a role in neurodevelopmental disorders, such as autism spectrum disorders. Understanding the science of the microbiome and its impact on human health is crucial for achieving optimal nutrition and holistic wellness. The composition and functioning of our microbiome are heavily influenced by our diet, with fiber and prebiotics playing a vital role in nurturing a healthy gut microbiome. A diet rich in fruits, vegetables, whole grains, and prebiotic-rich foods promotes the growth of beneficial bacteria, while a diet high in saturated fats and sugar disrupts the balance of the microbiome, leading to chronic inflammation and an increased risk of diseases. The microbiome-brain axis highlights the influence of the gut microbiome on mental health, underscoring the importance of a healthy microbiome for overall well-being. By making conscious choices about the foods we eat, we can optimize our microbiome for better health.

VI. THE EFFECTS OF PROCESSED FOODS ON THE MICROBIOME

Processed foods have become a predominant part of the modern diet, largely due to their convenience and long shelf life. The excessive consumption of processed foods has been associated with numerous negative health effects, including an altered microbiome. The microbiome refers to the diverse community of microorganisms that reside in the human body, particularly in the gut. These microorganisms play a crucial role in various physiological processes, such as digestion, immune function, and maintaining overall health. The consumption of processed foods has been shown to disrupt the delicate balance of the gut microbiome, leading to a multitude of detrimental effects on our health. One of the keyways in which processed foods impact the microbiome is by altering its diversity. A diverse and balanced microbiome is associated with optimal health, while a reduced diversity has been linked to various diseases, such as obesity, diabetes, and inflammatory bowel disease. Processed foods are typically low in fiber and high in refined sugars, unhealthy fats, and additives. These dietary components promote the growth of certain types of bacteria, such as Firmicutes, while discouraging the growth of beneficial bacteria, such as Bacteroidetes. This imbalance in the composition of the microbiome can lead to dysbiosis, a condition characterized by an overgrowth of harmful bacteria and a decrease in beneficial bacteria.

The consumption of processed foods can disrupt the integrity of the gut barrier, which is crucial for maintaining the health of the microbiome. The gut barrier acts as a protective layer between the gut microbiota and the rest of the body, preventing harmful substances from entering the bloodstream. The excessive consumption of processed foods, particularly those high in unhealthy fats and additives, can lead to the disruption of the gut barrier, allowing harmful bacteria and toxins to pass through and enter the bloodstream. This can trigger an immune response, leading to chronic inflammation and increasing the risk of various inflammatory diseases, such as irritable bowel syndrome and autoimmune disorders. In addition to altering the composition of the microbiome and compromising the gut barrier, processed foods can also influence the functionality of the microbiome. The gut microbiota plays a crucial role in the digestion and absorption of nutrients. The consumption of processed foods, which are often low in essential nutrients and high in unhealthy additives, can deprive the microbiome of the necessary nutrients it needs to function optimally. Certain additives commonly found in processed foods, such as emulsifiers and artificial sweeteners, have been shown to have detrimental effects on the microbiome. For example, studies have found that emulsifiers can alter the composition of the gut microbiota and promote inflammation, while artificial sweeteners have been shown to negatively affect glucose metabolism and disrupt the balance of the microbiome. The impact of processed foods on the microbiome extends beyond the gut, affecting other aspects of our health as well. Emerging research suggests that dysbiosis caused by the consumption of processed foods can influence mental health and cognitive function. The gut-brain axis, a bidirectional communication system between the gut and the brain, plays a crucial role in regulating mood and cognitive function. Disruptions in the gut microbiome, such as those caused by the consumption of processed foods, have been linked to an increased risk of mental health disorders, such as anxiety and depression, as well as neurodegenerative diseases, such as Alzheimer's disease. The excessive consumption of processed foods has a detrimental effect on the microbiome, impacting its diversity, integrity, functionality, and ultimately our overall health. The composition of processed foods, with their high content of unhealthy fats, refined sugars, and additives, disrupts the delicate balance of the microbiome, leading to dysbiosis and chronic inflammation. Processed foods compromise the integrity of the gut barrier, allowing harmful bacteria and toxins to enter the bloodstream, further exacerbating inflammation and increasing the risk of various inflammatory diseases. The consumption of processed foods deprives the microbiome of essential nutrients, impacting its functionality and the overall health of the individual. Emerging research suggests that dysbiosis caused by processed foods can influence mental health and cognitive function, further underscoring the importance of consuming a balanced and nutritious diet for optimal health. By understanding the effects of processed foods on the microbiome, individuals can make informed choices about their diet, promoting a diverse and balanced microbiome for improved overall health and wellness.

THE NEGATIVE IMPACT OF PROCESSED FOODS ON THE MICROBIOME

Processed foods have gained significant popularity in recent years, thanks to their convenience and appealing taste. Research has shown that these types of foods can have a negative impact on the microbiome. Processed foods are typically low in fiber and high in sugar, unhealthy fats, and artificial additives. These factors contribute to the disruption of the delicate balance of the microbial community in our gut, leading to a less diverse and less resilient microbiome.

One of the main reasons processed foods negatively affect the microbiome is their low fiber content. Fiber acts as a prebiotic, providing nourishment for the beneficial bacteria in our gut. When we consume processed foods that are stripped of fiber, it starves our gut microbes and hinders their ability to thrive. This leads to a decrease in the abundance of beneficial bacteria, such as Bifidobacterium and Lactobacillus, which are known for their role in supporting our immune system and promoting overall gut health. A lack of fiber intake from processed foods can result in constipation and other digestive issues, further compromising the health of our microbiome.

Processed foods are also notorious for their high sugar content. Excessive sugar consumption has been linked to various health problems, including obesity, type 2 diabetes, and cardiovascular diseases. In terms of the microbiome, studies have shown that a diet high in sugar can promote the growth of harmful bacteria, such as Clostridium difficile, while reducing the abundance of beneficial bacteria. This disrupts the balance of our gut microbiota and can lead to inflammation, a weakened immune system, and an increased susceptibility to infections. The fermentation of sugar by certain pathogenic bacteria produces harmful by-products, such as short-chain fatty acids, which can damage the intestinal barrier and contribute to gut inflammation.

Unhealthy fats are another component of processed foods that negatively impact the microbiome. Trans fats, for example, are commonly found in fried and processed foods and have been shown to alter the composition of the gut microbiota. Research suggests that consuming trans fats can increase the abundance of harmful bacteria, such as Bilophila wadsworthia, and decrease the levels of beneficial bacteria, including Bifidobacterium and Akkermansia muciniphila. This imbalance can lead to gut dysbiosis, a condition characterized by reduced microbial diversity and impaired gut function. Trans fats have been found to promote inflammation and insulin resistance, further compromising overall health. Artificial additives, which are prevalent in processed foods, also have a negative impact on the microbiome. These additives can include preservatives, colorings, flavor enhancers, and emulsifiers. While these substances are designed to improve the taste, texture, and shelf life of processed foods, they can disrupt the balance of our gut microbiota. Some additives have been shown to alter the composition of the microbial community and promote the growth of pathogenic bacteria. For example, emulsifiers like polysorbate 80 and carboxymethylcellulose have been found to induce gut inflammation and alter the gut barrier function in animal studies. These findings suggest that the consumption of processed foods containing artificial additives can contribute to gut dysbiosis and increase the risk of developing chronic inflammatory conditions, such as inflammatory bowel disease.

The negative impact of processed foods on the microbiome is a result of their low fiber content, high sugar and unhealthy fat content, as well as the presence of artificial additives. These factors disrupt the delicate balance of the gut microbial community and lead to a less diverse and less resilient microbiome. Consequently, individuals who consume processed foods regularly may experience digestive issues, weakened immune function, increased inflammation, and an elevated risk of chronic diseases. To promote optimal health and support a thriving microbiome, it is crucial to prioritize whole, unprocessed foods that are rich in fiber, promote beneficial bacteria, and avoid harmful additives.

ADDITIVES, PRESERVATIVES, AND ARTIFICIAL INGREDIENTS CAN DISRUPT THE MICROBIOME

There has been a growing concern about the potential negative effects of additives, preservatives, and artificial ingredients on our health, particularly on our gut microbiome. The gut microbiome is a complex community of trillions of microorganisms that reside in our digestive system and play a crucial role in maintaining our overall health. These microorganisms help with digestion, provide essential nutrients, support our immune system, and even affect our mental health. The consumption of processed foods that are high in additives, preservatives, and artificial ingredients has been shown to disrupt the delicate balance of these microorganisms, leading to a cascade of negative health effects. One of the major concerns with additives in our food supply is their potential to negatively impact the diversity and composition of our gut microbiome. Additives are substances that are added to food during processing to enhance its taste, texture, color, or shelf life. These include artificial sweeteners, flavor enhancers, emulsifiers, and stabilizers. While these additives may seem harmless, studies have shown that they can drastically alter the microbial communities in our gut.

For example, artificial sweeteners like aspartame and sucralose have been found to disrupt the balance of gut bacteria, leading to a decrease in beneficial bacteria and an increase in harmful ones. This disruption in the gut microbiome has been linked to a variety of health issues, including metabolic disorders, obesity, and even an increased risk of developing type 2 diabetes. Similarly, emulsifiers, which are commonly found in processed foods and baked goods, have also been shown to negatively impact the gut microbiome. These substances can alter the integrity of the intestinal barrier, leading to inflammation and increased permeability, commonly referred to as "leaky gut syndrome." This, in turn, can contribute to the development of chronic inflammatory conditions such as inflammatory bowel disease and autoimmune diseases. Preservatives, on the other hand, are substances added to food to prolong its shelf life and prevent spoilage. While preservatives are necessary to prevent foodborne illnesses and ensure the safety of our food supply, their excessive use can have detrimental effects on our gut microbiome. Common preservatives like sodium benzoate and potassium sorbate have been shown to have antimicrobial properties, meaning that they can kill or inhibit the growth of bacteria, both beneficial and harmful. This disruption in the balance of gut bacteria can have wide-ranging effects on our health, as these microorganisms play a crucial role in various physiological processes. Artificial ingredients, such as artificial flavors, colors, and additives, are often added to processed foods to make them more appealing and visually attractive. These artificial ingredients have been shown to have negative effects on the gut microbiome. For instance, artificial colors, such as tartrazine and red #40, have been associated with increased inflammation in the gut and alterations in gut microbiota composition. Similarly, artificial flavors, which are often derived from chemical compounds, can disrupt the delicate balance of the gut microbiome, contributing to gut dysbiosis and associated health issues. The consumption of foods high in additives, preservatives, and artificial ingredients can disrupt the delicate balance of our gut microbiome, leading to a multitude of negative health effects. These substances have been shown to alter the composition and diversity of our gut bacteria, leading to an increase in harmful bacteria and a decrease in beneficial ones. This imbalance in the gut microbiome has been linked to a variety of health issues, including metabolic disorders, obesity, chronic inflammation, and autoimmune diseases. It is crucial to prioritize whole, unprocessed foods that are free from these additives, preservatives, and artificial ingredients, in order to optimize our gut microbiome and promote overall health and wellness.

THE LONG-TERM CONSEQUENCES OF RELYING ON PROCESSED FOODS FOR NUTRITION

Processed foods have become a pervasive staple in the modern Western diet, offering convenience and affordability. The long-term consequences of relying on processed foods for nutrition can be detrimental to our overall health. One of the main concerns with processed foods is their high sugar content. Many processed foods are loaded with added sugars, which not only contribute to weight gain but also increase the risk of developing chronic diseases such as heart disease and type 2 diabetes. Excessive sugar consumption has been linked to an increased prevalence of obesity, insulin resistance, and metabolic syndrome. The high levels of refined carbohydrates found in processed foods can lead to rapid spikes in blood sugar levels, followed by crashes, which can leave individuals feeling lethargic and hungry, ultimately leading to overeating and weight gain.

In addition to their impact on weight and metabolic health, processed foods can have detrimental effects on the gut microbiome. The gut microbiome refers to the trillions of microorganisms that reside in our intestines, playing a crucial role in maintaining our overall health. Studies have shown that the consumption of processed foods can alter the composition and diversity of the gut microbiome, leading to a dysbiosis, or an imbalance in the microbial community. This dysbiosis has been associated with various health conditions, including inflammatory bowel disease, obesity, and metabolic disorders.

One of the reasons why processed foods negatively impact the gut microbiome is their lack of dietary fiber. Dietary fiber, found in whole grains, fruits, vegetables, and legumes, acts as a prebiotic, providing nourishment to the beneficial bacteria in our gut. Without sufficient dietary fiber, these beneficial bacteria cannot thrive, leading to a decline in their populations. This decline in beneficial bacteria can disrupt the delicate balance of the gut microbiome and contribute to the development of various health issues. Processed foods often contain artificial additives and preservatives, which can have harmful effects on the gut microbiome. These additives have been shown to alter the composition and function of the gut microbiome, leading to increased intestinal permeability, or leaky gut syndrome. When the intestinal barrier becomes compromised, harmful toxins and bacteria can enter the bloodstream, triggering inflammation and potentially contributing to the development of chronic diseases such as inflammatory bowel disease, autoimmune disorders, and even mental health conditions.

Another concern with relying on processed foods is their nutrient-poor nature. While they may be fortified with certain vitamins and minerals, processed foods are typically stripped of their natural nutrients during the refining and manufacturing processes. This nutrient depletion can lead to various deficiencies, such as those in essential vitamins and minerals like vitamin D, vitamin B12, calcium, and iron. These deficiencies can have far-reaching consequences on our health, leading to impaired immune function, decreased bone density, and anemia.

Processed foods are often high in unhealthy fats and low in healthy fats. The excessive consumption of unhealthy, saturated fats found in processed foods can contribute to the development of heart disease, while a lack of healthy fats, such as those found in fatty fish, avocados, and nuts, can deprive our bodies of essential omega-3 fatty acids and other beneficial compounds that are vital for brain health, cardiovascular health, and overall well-being. Relying on processed foods for nutrition can have numerous long-term consequences on our health. The high sugar content, lack of dietary fiber, presence of artificial additives, nutrient depletion, and imbalance of unhealthy fats all contribute to a host of chronic diseases and health conditions. To ensure optimal nutrition and promote a healthy gut microbiome, it is crucial to prioritize whole, unprocessed foods in our diets. By incorporating a variety of fruits, vegetables, whole grains, legumes, lean proteins, and healthy fats, we can support the health and diversity of our gut microbiome and ultimately improve our overall well-being.

There has been a growing interest in the science of the microbiome and its impact on human health. The microbiome refers to the trillions of microorganisms that reside within our bodies, particularly in our gut. These microorganisms play a crucial role in maintaining our overall health and well-being, influencing various aspects of our physiology, including our metabolism, immune system, and brain function. Understanding the microbiome and its relationship with our dietary choices is key to achieving optimal nutrition and holistic wellness.

One of the most significant ways in which the microbiome affects our health is through its involvement in the metabolism and digestion of food. The microorganisms in our gut break down complex carbohydrates, proteins, and fats that are otherwise indigestible by our own enzymes. They produce enzymes that can break down these compounds into smaller, more easily absorbable molecules, allowing our bodies to receive the necessary nutrients from our diet. In return, these microorganisms also benefit from the byproducts of their metabolism, such as short-chain fatty acids, which serve as a source of energy for both the gut microbiota and our own cells.

The microbiome has a profound influence on our immune system. Through various mechanisms, the microorganisms in our gut help educate and regulate our immune cells, teaching them to distinguish between harmless substances and potentially harmful pathogens. This interaction between the microbiome and the immune system is crucial for maintaining a healthy balance and preventing chronic inflammation, which has been implicated in the development of numerous diseases, including autoimmune disorders, allergies, and even mental health conditions. Recent research has shed light on the intricate connection between the microbiome and our brain. The gut-brain axis is a bidirectional communication network that allows the gut microbiota to communicate with our central nervous system. This communication occurs through chemical messengers, such as neurotransmitters and immune factors, which can influence brain function and behavior. For example, certain gut bacteria have been found to produce neurotransmitters like serotonin, a key regulator of mood, which suggests a link between the microbiome and mental health conditions like depression and anxiety. Understanding the microbiome's influence on the brain is crucial for developing new therapeutic approaches for conditions affecting mental well-being. Given the significant impact of the microbiome on our health, it is evident that our dietary choices can profoundly influence the composition and functioning of this complex ecosystem. Research has shown that a diet rich in dietary fiber, fruits, and vegetables promotes the growth of beneficial microorganisms in the gut. These plant-based foods are excellent sources of prebiotics, which serve as fuel for the growth of probiotics, beneficial bacteria that contribute to a healthy microbiome. Fermented foods, like yogurt and kimchi, are rich in probiotics and can introduce these beneficial microorganisms into our digestive system. A Western-style diet, characterized by high consumption of processed foods, added sugars, and saturated fats, has been shown to have detrimental effects on the microbiome. This type of diet is associated with a decrease in microbial diversity, with potentially harmful microorganisms becoming more dominant. This dysbiosis, or imbalance in the microbiome, has been linked to various health conditions, including obesity, type 2 diabetes, and inflammatory bowel diseases. Consequently, adopting a whole-food, plant-based diet can be a proactive approach to promote a healthy microbiome and prevent the development of these chronic diseases. Understanding the science of the microbiome and its impact on human health is essential for achieving optimal nutrition and holistic wellness. The microbiome plays a pivotal role in our metabolism, immune system, and brain function, influencing various aspects of our physiology. Dietary choices have a profound influence on the composition and functioning of the microbiome, with a plant-based, whole-food diet being associated with a healthy microbiome and improved overall health. By nourishing the microbiome through mindful dietary choices, we can embark on a transformative journey towards holistic wellness and improved quality of life.

VII. THE BENEFITS OF FIBER FOR THE MICROBIOME

One of the key components of optimal nutrition for the microbiome is fiber. Fiber is a type of carbohydrate that is found in plant-based foods, such as fruits, vegetables, whole grains, and legumes. It is not digestible by humans, but it serves as a valuable food source for the bacteria in our gut.

When fiber reaches the colon, it undergoes fermentation by the microbiota. This process results in the production of short-chain fatty acids (SCFAs), such as acetate, propionate, and butyrate. SCFAs are essential for maintaining a healthy gut and have been linked to numerous health benefits.

Firstly, SCFAs play a crucial role in maintaining the integrity of the gut barrier. The gut barrier acts as a protective barrier against harmful substances and bacteria that can potentially enter the bloodstream. SCFAs promote the production of mucin, a protective layer that lines the intestinal wall and helps prevent the invasion of pathogens. SCFAs enhance the production of tight junction proteins, which strengthen the connections between intestinal cells, further improving the integrity of the gut barrier. A compromised gut barrier has been associated with various intestinal disorders, such as inflammatory bowel disease (IBD) and irritable bowel syndrome (IBS).

SCFAs have anti-inflammatory properties. They have been shown to inhibit the production of pro-inflammatory cytokines, which are molecules that are responsible for promoting inflammation in the body. Chronic inflammation has been linked to the development of various chronic conditions, such as obesity, cardiovascular disease, and autoimmune diseases. By reducing inflammation, SCFAs can help prevent the onset of these serious health conditions. SCFAs have been found to play a role in regulating appetite and weight management. Butyrate, in particular, has been shown to increase the production of appetite-regulating hormones, such as peptide YY (PYY) and glucagon-like peptide-1 (GLP-1). These hormones help signal to the brain that we are full, thereby reducing our food intake. SCFAs have been shown to increase the expression of genes involved in fat oxidation, leading to increased energy expenditure and potential weight loss. In addition to the production of SCFAs, fiber consumption also promotes the growth of beneficial bacteria in the gut. Fiber acts as a prebiotic, providing nourishment for these beneficial bacteria. These bacteria help maintain a healthy balance of microorganisms in the gut, crowding out potentially harmful bacteria and promoting overall gut health. A diverse and well-balanced gut microbiota has been associated with improved immune function, reduced risk of infection, and protection against chronic diseases. Not only does fiber benefit the gut microbiome, but it also has a positive impact on other aspects of our health. For instance, a high-fiber diet has been shown to lower the risk of developing various chronic diseases, such as type 2 diabetes, cardiovascular disease, and certain types of cancer. Fiber helps regulate blood sugar levels by slowing down the absorption of glucose, preventing spikes in blood sugar. Fiber helps lower cholesterol levels by binding to bile acids in the gut and promoting their excretion. This reduces the amount of cholesterol that is recycled back into the bloodstream, leading to lower levels of LDL cholesterol, which is often referred to as "bad" cholesterol. Fiber plays a crucial role in promoting optimal nutrition for the microbiome. It serves as a valuable food source for the bacteria in our gut, promoting the production of beneficial short-chain fatty acids and the growth of beneficial bacteria. These SCFAs have a wide range of health benefits, including maintaining the integrity of the gut barrier, reducing inflammation, regulating appetite and weight man-agement, and promoting overall gut health. Fiber consumption has been associated with a reduced risk of developing chronic diseases, such as type 2 diabetes, cardiovascular disease, and certain types of cancer. Incorporating fiber-rich foods into our diet is essential for improving our microbiome and achieving holistic wellness.

THE ROLE OF FIBER IN PROMOTING A HEALTHY MICROBIOME

Fiber plays a crucial role in promoting a healthy microbiome, which is essential for optimal nutrition and overall wellness. The human microbiome refers to the trillions of microorganisms that inhabit our bodies, particularly the gut. These microorganisms, including bacteria, fungi, viruses, and archaea, play a vital role in maintaining our health by aiding in digestion, nutrient absorption, immune function, and even influencing our mental health. The composition and diversity of the microbiome greatly impact its functionality, and dietary fiber plays a significant role in shaping the microbiome's composition. Fiber refers to the indigestible components of plant foods that pass through the digestive system largely intact. It encompasses two types: soluble fiber, which dissolves in water, and insoluble fiber, which does not. Both types of fiber are essential for a healthy microbiome. Soluble fiber is fermented by the bacteria in the gut, resulting in the production of short-chain fatty acids (SCFAs). SCFAs, particularly butyrate, acetate, and propionate, act as an energy source for the cells that line the gut and have been associated with numerous health benefits. These SCFAs provide nourishment to the colonocytes, or colon cells, promoting their growth and strengthening the integrity of the gut barrier. A healthy gut barrier is essential in preventing the translocation of harmful substances, such as bacteria and toxins, from the gut into the bloodstream, reducing the risk of systemic inflammation and chronic diseases. SCFAs have been shown to interact with and modulate the immune system, leading to reduced in-flammation and improved immune function. This interaction helps prevent the development of autoimmune disorders, aller-gies, and other immune-related conditions.

Insoluble fiber, on the other hand, acts as a prebiotic, providing nourishment for beneficial gut bacteria. Prebiotics are substanc-es that selectively stimulate the growth of beneficial bacteria in the gut. By promoting the growth of these beneficial bacteria, insoluble fiber helps maintain a healthy balance of gut microbi-ota and supports optimal digestion and nutrient absorption. Insoluble fiber also adds bulk to the stool, preventing constipa-tion and promoting regular bowel movements. This, in turn, helps remove waste and toxins from the body efficiently, ensur-ing the healthy elimination of harmful substances.

Fiber-rich foods, particularly plant-based foods, are generally associated with a high nutrient density. Consuming a variety of fiber-rich foods provides essential vitamins, minerals, antioxi-dants, and phytochemicals necessary for optimal health. These nutrients not only support the growth and function of the micro-biome but also contribute to overall physical and mental well-ness. Research has consistently shown that populations with high-fiber diets have lower rates of chronic diseases, including cardiovascular disease, type 2 diabetes, obesity, and certain cancers. The diversity of the gut microbiome has been linked to reduced obesity and improved metabolic health. Fiber intake, especially soluble fiber, promotes the growth of beneficial bac-teria associated with a lean phenotype and the metabolism of dietary fiber, leading to better weight management and meta-bolic regulation. Fiber plays a critical role in promoting a healthy microbiome, which is crucial for optimal nutrition and overall wellness. Soluble fiber acts as a source of energy for gut cells, strengthening the gut barrier and modulating the immune system, thereby reducing inflammation and preventing chronic diseases. Insoluble fiber acts as a prebiotic, stimulating the growth of beneficial gut bacteria, supporting digestion, and preventing constipation. Fiber-rich foods, being nutrient-dense, provide essential vitamins, minerals, antioxidants, and phytochemicals necessary for overall health. Consuming a high-fiber diet has been consistently associated with lower rates of chronic diseases and improved metabolic health.

Incorporating an adequate amount of fiber, both soluble and insoluble, through a diverse range of plant-based foods, is essential for promoting a healthy microbiome and achieving holistic wellness.

THE DIFFERENT TYPES OF FIBER AND THEIR SPECIFIC EFFECTS ON THE MICROBIOME

There are several different types of fiber that can have specific effects on the microbiome. Soluble fiber, for example, is a type of fiber that dissolves in water and forms a gel-like substance in the digestive tract. This type of fiber is found in foods such as oats, barley, beans, lentils, and some fruits and vegetables. Soluble fiber is particularly beneficial for the microbiome because it acts as a prebiotic, providing nourishment for beneficial bacteria. These bacteria ferment soluble fiber and produce short-chain fatty acids (SCFAs), such as acetate, propionate, and butyrate, which are important for gut health. SCFAs provide energy for the cells lining the colon, promote the growth of beneficial bacteria, and have anti-inflammatory effects. Soluble fiber can help regulate blood sugar levels and lower cholesterol levels.

Another type of fiber that can promote a healthy microbiome is insoluble fiber. This type of fiber does not dissolve in water and adds bulk to the stool, which helps to prevent constipation and promote regular bowel movements. Insoluble fiber can be found in whole grains, nuts, seeds, and the skins of fruits and vegetables. Although insoluble fiber does not provide nourishment for the microbiome in the same way that soluble fiber does, it still plays an important role in maintaining a healthy gut. By adding bulk to the stool, insoluble fiber helps to promote the growth of beneficial bacteria and prevent the overgrowth of harmful bacteria. It also helps to keep the digestive system moving smoothly, reducing the risk of developing conditions such as diverticulosis and colorectal cancer. Resistant starch is another type of fiber that has specific effects on the microbiome. This type of fiber is not broken down and absorbed in the small intestine like other starches. Instead, it travels to the large intestine, where it is fermented by beneficial bacteria. Resistant starch can be found in foods such as undercooked potatoes, green bananas, and legumes. The fermentation of resistant starch produces SCFAs, similar to the fermentation of soluble fiber. These SCFAs provide fuel for the cells lining the colon and have been shown to have numerous health benefits, including reducing inflammation and improving insulin sensitivity. In addition to these types of fiber, there are also prebiotics, which are a type of fiber that specifically nourishes beneficial bacteria in the gut. Prebiotics can be found in foods such as Jerusalem artichokes, chicory root, garlic, onions, and leeks. These foods contain nondigestible carbohydrates that pass through the upper gastrointestinal tract and reach the colon intact, where they are fermented by beneficial bacteria. By providing nourishment for beneficial bacteria, prebiotics can help to promote a healthy balance of bacteria in the gut and improve overall gut health. They have been shown to have numerous health benefits, including improving digestion, boosting the immune system, and reducing the risk of developing chronic diseases. The types of fiber that we consume can have specific effects on the microbiome. Soluble fiber acts as a prebiotic, nourishing beneficial bacteria and promoting the production of SCFAs, which have numerous health benefits. Insoluble fiber adds bulk to the stool and helps to prevent constipation, while also promoting the growth of beneficial bacteria. Resistant starch, another type of fiber, is fermented by beneficial bacteria in the colon, producing SCFAs and providing a range of health benefits. Prebiotics specifically nourish beneficial bacteria and contribute to a healthy balance of bacteria in the gut. By understanding the specific effects of different types of fiber on the microbiome, we can make informed dietary choices that promote optimal nutrition and improve our overall health and wellness.

THE DIETARY SOURCES OF FIBER AND HOW TO INCORPORATE IT INTO A BALANCED DIET

Fiber is an essential component of a balanced diet and plays a crucial role in maintaining digestive health. It is a type of carbohydrate that cannot be broken down by the enzymes in our digestive system, meaning it passes through our intestines intact. There are two main types of dietary fiber: soluble fiber and insoluble fiber. Soluble fiber dissolves in water to form a gel-like substance in the intestines and is found in foods such as oats, beans, and certain fruits and vegetables. Insoluble fiber does not dissolve in water and adds bulk to the stool, promoting regular bowel movements. It is commonly found in foods like whole grains, nuts, and certain vegetables. Both types of fiber are beneficial for our health and should be incorporated into our diet in adequate amounts. Many plant-based foods are excellent sources of fiber. Whole grains, such as brown rice, quinoa, and whole wheat products, are packed with fiber and provide other important nutrients as well. Incorporating these grains into our meals is a simple way to increase our fiber intake. Legumes, including beans, lentils, and chickpeas, are also high in fiber. By adding them to soups, stews, salads, and side dishes, we can easily boost our daily fiber intake. Fruits and vegetables are another great source of fiber. Berries, such as raspberries and blueberries, are particularly high in fiber and can be enjoyed as a snack or added to smoothies and yogurt. Leafy greens, like spinach and kale, are not only rich in fiber but also provide numerous vitamins and minerals. Including a variety of fruits and vegetables in our daily meals ensures a good intake of fiber. Incorporating fiber into a balanced diet can be done by making small and gradual changes to our eating habits. One easy way to increase fiber intake is to choose whole grain bread and pasta instead of refined white varieties. The whole grains retain more of their natural fiber content, making them a healthier choice. Another simple step is to opt for brown rice instead of white rice, as brown rice contains more fiber due to the presence of the grain's bran and germ. By gradually replacing refined grains with whole grains in our meals, we can significantly increase our daily fiber intake without sacrificing taste or enjoyment. Including a serving of legumes, such as beans or lentils, in our meals a few times a week can also contribute to our fiber intake. They can be easily incorporated into soups, stews, and salads or used as a protein-rich base for vegetarian meals. Getting enough fiber is not just about the foods we eat but also how we prepare them. Cooking fruits and vegetables can sometimes reduce their fiber content, so it is advisable to consume them in their raw or lightly cooked forms whenever possible. Alternatively, steaming or boiling them for a short period of time preserves more of their fiber content compared to long cooking methods. Keeping the skin on fruits and vegetables whenever possible also increases our fiber intake. For example, leaving the skin on potatoes and apples adds more fiber to our diet. By being aware of the preparation methods we use, we can ensure maximum fiber retention in our meals.

Fiber is an important component of a balanced diet and plays a crucial role in maintaining digestive health. Incorporating fiber into our diet can be achieved by consuming foods such as whole grains, legumes, fruits, and vegetables. Making small and gradual changes like choosing whole grain options, including leg-umes in our meals, and consuming fruits and vegetables in their raw or lightly cooked forms can significantly increase our fiber intake. By paying attention to our fiber consumption and mak-ing conscious choices, we can promote optimal nutrition and overall well-being. The microbiome, a diverse community of microorganisms that reside in the human body, has sparked great interest among scientists in recent years. This intricate ecosystem, primarily found in the gastrointestinal tract, plays a crucial role in maintaining our overall health and well-being. Collectively, these microorganisms weigh about three pounds, and their genetic material outnumbers our own by a startling ratio of ten to one. Exploring the science of the microbiome and understanding how it is influenced by our dietary choices is key to achieving optimal nutrition and overall wellness.

To comprehend the significance of the microbiome, one must first appreciate its complexity. While bacteria are prominent members of this community, it also includes viruses, fungi, and other microorganisms. These microbes are not simply passen-gers within our bodies; they actively engage in significant physi-ological processes. For example, they aid in the digestion and absorption of nutrients, produce vitamins, and regulate our im-mune system. The microbiome helps protect us from harmful pathogens, serving as a barrier to potential infections.

Understanding the factors that shape the composition of the microbiome is crucial in improving our health. One significant influence is the foods we consume. Our diet directly impacts the diversity and functionality of our gut microbiota. A diet consist-ing of whole, minimally processed foods, rich in fruits, vegeta-bles, and whole grains, is associated with a more diverse and beneficial microbiome. These plant-based foods provide the necessary nutrients for the growth and survival of beneficial bacteria, promoting a balanced microbial community. In contrast, a diet high in processed foods, refined sugars, and unhealthy fats is linked to a less diverse microbiome, with an overgrowth of potentially harmful bacteria.

In addition to the overall composition of the microbiome, the foods we eat also affect the production of specific metabolites, or small molecules, by the gut bacteria. These metabolites have far-reaching effects on our health. For instance, short-chain fatty acids (SCFAs), like butyrate, are produced by certain bacteria during the fermentation of dietary fiber. SCFAs have been shown to have anti-inflammatory properties and promote a healthy intestinal lining. A lack of dietary fiber and subsequent decrease in SCFA production may contribute to chronic inflammation and the development of conditions like inflammatory bowel disease. The influence of the microbiome extends beyond the gastrointestinal tract. It has been implicated in numerous diseases and conditions, including obesity, type 2 diabetes, cardiovascular disease, and mental health disorders. For example, studies have shown that individuals with obesity have a distinct microbial profile compared to lean individuals. The abundance of certain bacteria species can affect the efficiency of energy extraction from food, leading to weight gain or difficulty in losing weight. The microbiome has been found to have an impact on hormone regulation, including insulin sensitivity, which plays a significant role in the development of type 2 diabetes. The emerging field of research on the microbiome has provided valuable insights into potential therapeutic interventions. By understanding the interactions between the microbiota and host, interventions aimed at modulating the microbiome can be developed. Probiotics, live microorganisms that confer health benefits when consumed, have gained popularity as a means to improve gut health. They can restore a disrupted microbial community and may alleviate certain digestive disorders. Prebiotics, on the other hand, are indigestible fibers that stimulate the growth of beneficial bacteria. They can be found in foods such as onions, garlic, and bananas and can be used as an additional tool to promote microbial diversity. The microbiome plays a significant role in our overall health and well-being. The foods we consume directly influence the composition and functionality of our gut microbiota. By adopting a diet rich in whole, plant-based foods, we can support the growth of beneficial bacteria and promote a diverse microbial community. This, in turn, may have profound effects on our immune system, metabolism, and overall health. As the importance of the microbiome continues to be unraveled, further research may lead to novel insights into the prevention and treatment of various diseases.

VIII. THE GUT-BRAIN AXIS: UNDERSTANDING THE CONNECTION

The gut-brain axis refers to the bidirectional communication between the gut and the brain, highlighting the intricate relationship between the two. Research has shown that the gut microbiota can influence brain function and behavior through various mechanisms. One of the key players in this complex interaction is the vagus nerve, which serves as a direct communication pathway between the gut and the brain. The vagus nerve allows for the transmission of signals from the gut microbiota to the brain, providing valuable information about the gut's state and facilitating the regulation of brain function. This bidirectional communication is further supported by the production of neurotransmitters in the gut, such as serotonin and γ-aminobutyric acid (GABA), which can travel to the brain and affect mood, cognition, and behavior. The gut-brain axis has been implicated in several neurological disorders, including anxiety, depression, and autism spectrum disorders. Studies have shown that alterations in gut microbiota composition and function can disrupt the delicate balance of the gut-brain axis, leading to the development or exacerbation of these disorders. For example, individuals with depression often exhibit an imbalance in their gut microbiota, characterized by a decrease in beneficial bacteria and an increase in opportunistic pathogens. This dysbiosis can trigger inflammatory responses and alter neurotransmitter production, ultimately affecting mood and behavior. Alterations in the gut-brain axis have been observed in individuals with autism spectrum disorders, suggesting a potential role for the gut microbiota in the pathogenesis of these conditions.

Understanding the gut-brain axis is crucial for optimizing our nutrition and overall health. By nourishing our gut microbiota, we can promote a healthy gut-brain axis and support optimal brain function and mental well-being. One way to achieve this is through the consumption of prebiotic and probiotic-rich foods.

Prebiotics are dietary fibers that serve as food for our gut microbiota, promoting the growth and activity of beneficial bacteria. Foods rich in prebiotics include garlic, onions, asparagus, and bananas. Probiotics, on the other hand, are live bacteria that can directly supplement our gut microbiota. Fermented foods such as yogurt, sauerkraut, and kimchi are excellent sources of probiotics. In addition to modulating the gut-brain axis through diet, lifestyle factors also play a significant role in maintaining a healthy gut microbiota and optimizing the gut-brain connection. Regular physical activity has been shown to enhance gut microbial diversity and promote the production of beneficial compounds. Exercise can stimulate the release of short-chain fatty acids, which provide energy for the cells lining the gut and have anti-inflammatory effects. Stress management techniques, such as Mindfulness meditation and yoga, have been found to positively impact the gut-brain axis. Chronic stress can impair gut barrier function and alter gut microbiota composition, further highlighting the importance of stress reduction in maintaining a healthy gut-brain connection.

The gut-brain axis represents a complex and dynamic connection between the gut and the brain. The bidirectional communication between these two entities is mediated by the vagus nerve and the production of neurotransmitters in the gut. Alterations in gut microbiota composition and function can disrupt this connection and contribute to the development or exacerbation of neurological disorders. By nurturing our gut microbiota through diet and lifestyle interventions, we can optimize the gut-brain axis and promote optimal brain function and mental well-being. Prebiotic and probiotic-rich foods, regular physical activity, and stress management techniques all play a vital role in maintaining a healthy gut-brain connection. By understanding and harnessing the power of the gut-brain axis, we can unlock new strategies for improving our health and well-being.

THE RELATIONSHIP BETWEEN THE GUT MICROBIOME AND BRAIN HEALTH

The relationship between the gut microbiome and brain health is a topic of growing interest and research in the field of microbiology. It is now widely recognized that the gut microbiome, the collection of microorganisms that inhabit the gastrointestinal tract, plays a crucial role in maintaining overall health and well-being. Recent studies have also shown that the gut microbiome has a direct impact on brain health and function.

One of the ways in which the gut microbiome influences brain health is through the production of neurotransmitters. Neurotransmitters are chemicals that transmit signals in the brain, and they play a vital role in regulating mood, cognition, and behavior. Interestingly, many of these neurotransmitters, such as serotonin and dopamine, are actually produced in the gut. In fact, research has shown that a significant portion of serotonin, often referred to as the "feel-good" neurotransmitter, is produced by bacteria in the gut. This suggests that the composition of the gut microbiome can have a direct impact on the levels of neurotransmitters in the brain, and consequently, on mental health and well-being. The gut microbiome is also involved in the production and regulation of other molecules that can influence brain function. For example, the gut microbiome produces short-chain fatty acids (SCFAs), which are byproducts of the fermentation of dietary fiber by gut bacteria. SCFAs have been shown to have neuroprotective and anti-inflammatory effects in the brain. They can also act as a source of energy for brain cells, and they have been implicated in the regulation of mood and cognition. Research has also shown that alterations in the gut microbiome can lead to dysregulation of the production of SCFAs, which may contribute to the development of neurological disorders, such as depression and anxiety.

In addition to the production of neurotransmitters and other molecules, the gut microbiome can also influence brain health through its interaction with the immune system. The gut is home to a large number of immune cells, which are responsible for defending against harmful pathogens. These immune cells also play a role in regulating inflammation in the body, including in the brain. Emerging research has shown that alterations in the gut microbiome can lead to an imbalance in the immune response, resulting in chronic inflammation. This chronic inflammation has been linked to the development of neurodegenerative diseases, such as Alzheimer's disease, as well as mood disorders. Another way in which the gut microbiome can impact brain health is through the gut-brain axis, a bidirectional communication system between the gut and the brain. This communication occurs through various mechanisms, including the release of signaling molecules and the activation of neural pathways. The gut-brain axis is thought to play a crucial role in regulating mood, stress response, and cognitive function. Research has shown that alterations in the gut microbiome can disrupt the gut-brain axis, leading to dysregulation of these processes. For example, studies have shown that mice raised without gut bacteria exhibit altered stress responses and increased risk of anxiety-like behavior. The relationship between the gut microbiome and brain health is complex and multifaceted. It involves the production of neurotransmitters and other molecules that can directly influence brain function, as well as the regulation of the immune response and the gut-brain axis. Understanding this relationship is crucial for developing strategies to promote optimal brain health and prevent the development of neurological and psychiatric disorders. As research in this field continues to advance, it is becoming increasingly clear that a holistic approach to health, which includes nurturing a diverse and healthy gut microbiome through proper nutrition, is essential for promoting overall well-being and cognitive function.

THE COMMUNICATION PATHWAY BETWEEN THE GUT AND THE BRAIN

The communication pathway between the gut and the brain plays a crucial role in maintaining overall health and well-being. This bidirectional communication system, known as the gut-brain axis, involves intricate interactions between the gastrointestinal tract and the central nervous system. It is facilitated by a complex network of neurons, hormones, immune cells, and chemical messengers. The gut is lined with millions of nerve cells, known as the enteric nervous system, which can function independently from the brain. This enteric nervous system is often referred to as the "second brain" due to its ability to control various digestive functions, such as the movement of food, nutrient absorption, and hormone secretion. The gut is home to trillions of microorganisms, collectively known as the gut microbiota, which further contribute to the communication pathway between the gut and the brain. One of the key mechanisms through which the gut communicates with the brain is the release of signaling molecules and neurotransmitters. For instance, the gut microbiota can produce various neurotransmitters, such as serotonin, dopamine, and gamma-aminobutyric acid (GABA), which are known to influence mood, emotions, and behavior. Serotonin, often referred to as the "feel-good" neurotransmitter, is primarily produced in the gut and plays a crucial role in regulating mood, sleep, and appetite. Approximately 90% of serotonin in the body is found in the gut, highlighting the significant contribution of the gut microbiota in serotonin production. Dysregulation of serotonin levels has been implicated in various mental health disorders, such as depression and anxiety. In addition to neurotransmitters, the gut microbiota can also produce metabolites that can directly or indirectly influence brain function. Short-chain fatty acids (SCFAs), such as acetate, propionate, and butyrate, are the primary metabolites produced by gut bacteria during the fermentation process of dietary fibers. SCFAs can cross the blood-brain barrier and enter the central nervous system, where they can modulate neural activity and promote the production of neurotrophic factors, which are vital for the growth and maintenance of neurons. These metabolites have been shown to have anti-inflammatory and neuroprotective effects on the brain, and their dysregulation has been linked to neurodevelopmental and neurodegenerative disorders. Another important aspect of the gut-brain axis is the role of the immune system in mediating communication between the gut and the brain. The gut is equipped with a highly specialized immune system that protects against harmful pathogens while maintaining a symbiotic relationship with beneficial microbes. The gut microbiota plays a crucial role in the development and maturation of the immune system, particularly through the production of immunoglobulins and the regulation of immune cell function. Immune cells, such as T cells and macrophages, can produce signaling molecules, known as cytokines, in response to the presence of pathogens or alterations in the gut microbiota. These cytokines can travel to the brain through various routes, such as the bloodstream, vagus nerve, or specialized immune cells, and interact with neural circuits involved in mood, cognition, and behavior. The dysregulation of this immune communication has been implicated in the pathophysiology of various neuropsychiatric disorders, including depression, schizophrenia, and autism spectrum disorders.

The gut microbiota can influence the communication pathway between the gut and the brain through the regulation of the intestinal barrier function. The gut barrier consists of a single layer of cells that line the intestine and serve as a protective barrier against harmful substances, such as toxins and pathogens. The gut microbiota plays a crucial role in maintaining the integrity and function of the gut barrier by producing various compounds, such as mucins, antimicrobial peptides, and tight junction proteins. Disruption of the gut barrier, often referred to as "leaky gut," can lead to the influx of harmful substances into the bloodstream, triggering an immune response and inflammation. This chronic inflammation can then affect the neural circuits involved in the gut-brain axis, leading to various neurological and psychiatric symptoms. Conversely, a healthy and diverse gut microbiota has been associated with a more robust and resilient gut barrier, thus promoting a healthy gut-brain communication. The communication pathway between the gut and the brain plays a critical role in maintaining optimal health and well-being. The bidirectional communication system, mediated by the gut-brain axis, involves complex interactions between the enteric nervous system, gut microbiota, neurotransmitters, metabolites, immune cells, and chemical messengers. Dysregulation of this communication pathway has been implicated in various neurological and psychiatric disorders. Thus, understanding the intricate relationship between the gut and the brain can provide valuable insights into the development of therapeutic interventions targeting the gut microbiome to improve overall health and well-being.

NUTRITION CAN IMPACT BOTH THE GUT AND THE BRAIN FOR OPTIMAL MENTAL HEALTH

The intricate relationship between nutrition, gut health, and mental well-being cannot be overstated. Recent research has shed light on the important role that our gut microbiome plays in regulating brain health and function. The gut-brain axis, a bidirectional communication pathway, allows for communication between the gut microbiota and the central nervous system. This communication occurs through various mechanisms, including the release of neurotransmitters, hormones, and metabolites, which can directly impact our mental health.

Nutrition plays a crucial role in shaping the composition and diversity of our gut microbiota. A diet rich in fiber, prebiotics, and probiotics can promote the growth of beneficial bacteria in the gut, leading to a healthier microbiome. A diet high in saturated fats, sugars, and processed foods can disrupt the balance of gut bacteria, leading to dysbiosis, inflammation, and an increased risk of mental health disorders.

One way that nutrition influences the gut-brain axis is through the production of neurotransmitters. Serotonin, a neurotransmitter commonly associated with mood regulation, is primarily produced in the gut. The gut microbiota plays a key role in serotonin production, as certain strains of bacteria produce enzymes required for its synthesis. A healthy gut microbiome can therefore contribute to optimal serotonin levels and improved mental well-being. An imbalanced gut microbiota, as seen in conditions such as irritable bowel syndrome (IBS) or inflammatory bowel disease (IBD), has been associated with lower serotonin levels and an increased risk of depressive symptoms. Nutrition can impact the gut-brain axis by influencing the integrity of the gut barrier. The gut barrier serves as a protective barrier between the gut lumen and the bloodstream, preventing the entry of harmful substances and toxins. A healthy gut barrier is crucial for maintaining a balanced immune response and preventing systemic inflammation. Poor nutrition, such as a diet high in processed foods, can compromise the integrity of the gut barrier, leading to increased gut permeability, or leaky gut syndrome. This can allow harmful substances, such as bacteria and toxins, to enter the bloodstream, triggering an immune response and inflammation. Chronic inflammation has been linked to various mental health conditions, including depression and anxiety. In addition to its effects on the gut microbiota and gut barrier, nutrition can directly impact brain health and function. The brain requires a constant supply of nutrients, including vitamins, minerals, and fatty acids, to function optimally. A diet rich in nutrient-dense foods, such as fruits, vegetables, whole grains, and lean proteins, can provide the necessary nutrients for proper brain function. A diet lacking in essential nutrients, such as a diet high in processed foods, can deprive the brain of the necessary building blocks for neurotransmitter synthesis and overall brain health. One nutrient that has garnered significant attention for its role in brain health is omega-3 fatty acids. Omega-3 fatty acids, particularly eicosapentaenoic acid (EPA) and docosahexaenoic acid (DHA), are essential for brain development and function. These fatty acids are found abundantly in fatty fish, such as salmon and mackerel, as well as in walnuts and flaxseeds. Studies have shown that individuals with higher intakes of omega-3 fatty acids have a reduced risk of depression and cognitive decline. Nutrition plays a critical role in shaping the gut microbiota and maintaining optimal brain health. A diet rich in fiber, prebiotics, and probiotics can promote a healthy gut microbiome, while a diet high in saturated fats, sugars, and processed foods can disrupt the gut microbiota, leading to dysbiosis and an increased risk of mental health disorders. Nutrition also influences the gut-brain axis through the production of neurotransmitters and the integrity of the gut barrier. Specific nutrients, such as omega-3 fatty acids, have been shown to have a direct impact on brain health and function. By understanding the intricate relationship between nutrition, the gut microbiome, and mental health, we can harness the power of optimal nutrition to improve our overall well-being.

The importance of understanding the microbiome and its impact on human health cannot be overstated. The microbiome refers to the trillions of microorganisms that reside within and on our bodies, primarily in the gastrointestinal tract. These microorganisms, including bacteria, fungi, viruses, and other archaea, play a crucial role in maintaining our overall health and wellbeing. Recent advancements in technology have allowed scientists to study the microbiome in greater depth, providing valuable insights into its complex interactions with our bodies and the influence it has on various aspects of our health. One area of particular interest is the connection between the microbiome and nutrition, as the foods we eat have a profound impact on the composition and function of our microbiomes. Understanding this relationship is essential for achieving optimal nutrition and promoting holistic wellness. The composition of our microbiome is influenced by various factors, including genetics, environment, and most significantly, diet. Studies have shown that individuals who consume a diverse range of plant-based foods, rich in fiber, have a more diverse and beneficial microbiome compared to those with a diet dominated by processed foods and animal products. This diversity is crucial because it provides a greater number and variety of microorganisms that perform vital functions, such as digesting dietary fiber, producing essential vitamins, and modulating immune responses.

One key aspect of optimal nutrition is the consumption of prebiotics, which are dietary fibers that serve as food for the beneficial bacteria in our gut. Prebiotics are found in a variety of foods, including fruits, vegetables, whole grains, and legumes. When we consume these foods, the prebiotics they contain pass through our digestive system undigested until they reach the colon, where they are fermented by specific bacteria. This fermentation process produces short-chain fatty acids, such as butyrate, acetate, and propionate, which provide nourishment for the cells lining our colon and have been associated with numerous health benefits. The consumption of probiotics, which are live microorganisms that confer a health benefit when consumed, can also play a role in optimizing our microbiome. Probiotics are found in fermented foods like yogurt, kefir, sauerkraut, and tempeh. These foods contain live cultures of specific bacteria or yeasts that can establish themselves in our gut and contribute to the diversity and balance of our microbiome. Research has shown that probiotics can help regulate bowel movements, improve digestion, enhance immune function, and even reduce the risk of certain diseases, such as diarrhea, inflammatory bowel disease, and allergies.

In addition to prebiotics and probiotics, certain nutrients and phytochemicals found in specific foods have been identified as beneficial for our microbiome. For example, polyphenols, which are naturally occurring compounds found in fruits, vegetables, nuts, and seeds, possess potent antioxidant and anti-inflammatory properties that can positively affect the composition and activity of our gut bacteria. Resveratrol, a polyphenol abundant in grapes and red wine, is known to promote the growth of beneficial bacteria and inhibit the growth of harmful ones. Other polyphenols, like quercetin in onions and epicatechin in cocoa, have similar effects. Omega-3 fatty acids, primarily found in fatty fish, walnuts, flaxseeds, and chia seeds, have been shown to support a healthy microbiome. These essential fatty acids help reduce inflammation in the gut and promote the growth of beneficial bacteria such as Bifidobacterium and Lactobacillus. A diet high in saturated fats, commonly found in processed foods and animal products, has been associated with an unfavorable shift in the composition of the microbiome, leading to increased inflammation and a higher risk of chronic diseases. The microbiome plays a crucial role in maintaining our health and wellbeing. By understanding the intricate relationship between the microbiome and nutrition, we can make informed dietary choices to optimize our microbiomes and promote holistic wellness. Consuming a diverse range of plant-based foods, rich in prebiotics and probiotics, can enhance the composition and function of our microbiome. Incorporating foods rich in polyphenols and omega-3 fatty acids can further support a healthy microbiome and reduce the risk of chronic disease. By prioritizing optimal nutrition and nurturing our microbiomes, we can take a significant step towards better health and wellbeing.

IX. THE ROLE OF NUTRIGENOMICS IN PERSONALIZED NUTRITION

Advances in the field of nutrigenomics have revolutionized the concept of personalized nutrition, recognizing that each individual possesses a unique genetic makeup that influences how they respond to different nutrients in their diet. Nutrigenomics explores the complex interactions between genes, the environment, and dietary factors, with the aim of tailoring dietary recommendations to match an individual's genetic profile. By uncovering the specific genetic variations present in an individual, nutrigenomics can provide valuable insights into their nutritional requirements, allowing for the development of personalized dietary plans that optimize health and well-being.

One of the key areas where nutrigenomics is making significant strides is in the understanding of how genetic variations influence an individual's response to specific nutrients. For instance, certain genetic variations can affect how efficiently an individual metabolizes carbohydrates, fats, or proteins, leading to variations in how different individuals respond to these macronutrients. Through the identification of these genetic variants, nutrigenomics can inform personalized dietary recommendations, guiding individuals towards a diet that is optimized for their unique genetic makeup. This has important implications for weight management, as individuals with certain genetic variations may benefit from specific dietary approaches that are tailored to their metabolism. Nutrigenomics also sheds light on how genetic variations influence an individual's susceptibility to certain chronic diseases. By analyzing an individual's genetic profile, researchers can identify gene variants that are associated with an increased risk of developing conditions such as cardiovascular disease, diabetes, or certain types of cancer. Armed with this knowledge, nutrigenomics can guide individuals towards dietary choices that mitigate their risk of developing these diseases. For example, individuals with a genetic predisposition to heart disease may benefit from following a diet that is low in saturated fats and cholesterol, while those with a heightened risk of diabetes may be advised to consume a diet that is low in simple sugars and high in fiber. By leveraging the insights gained from nutrigenomics, personalized nutrition plans can be developed to not only optimize health outcomes but also prevent the onset of chronic diseases. Another aspect of nutrigenomics that holds great promise is its ability to uncover the mechanisms by which nutrients interact with genes and influence gene expression. The field of nutrigenomics has demonstrated that diet can have a significant impact on gene expression, with certain nutrients acting as either activators or inhibitors of specific genes. This has important implications for the regulation of gene expression, as it suggests that dietary choices can potentially modulate the activity of genes that influence disease susceptibility and overall health. For instance, certain nutrients have been found to influence the expression of genes involved in inflammation, oxidative stress, and DNA repair, all of which play a crucial role in disease development. By optimizing dietary choices to promote favorable gene expression patterns, nutrigenomics has the potential to unlock new strategies for disease prevention and health promotion.

Nutrigenomics represents a groundbreaking field of research

that combines genetics, nutrition, and personalized medicine. By uncovering the intricate interactions between genes, the environment, and dietary factors, nutrigenomics provides valuable insights into the specific nutritional requirements of individuals. This knowledge can then be used to develop personalized dietary plans that optimize health outcomes and prevent the onset of chronic diseases. Nutrigenomics also offers insights into how nutrients interact with genes and influence gene expression, opening up new avenues for disease prevention and health promotion. As our understanding of the role of genetics in nutrition continues to evolve, nutrigenomics promises to transform the way we approach nutrition, tailoring dietary recommendations to match an individual's unique genetic profile for optimal health and well-being.

THE FIELD OF NUTRIGENOMICS AND ITS RELEVANCE TO OPTIMAL NUTRITION

Nutrigenomics is a rapidly emerging field that studies the interaction between our genes and the food we consume, with the aim of understanding how nutrition can affect our health on a molecular level. The field of nutrigenomics goes beyond the traditional focus of nutrition, which is primarily concerned with the macro and micronutrient content of foods. Instead, it delves into the intricate relationship between our genetic makeup and the nutrients we consume, and how this interaction can influence gene expression and cellular processes. This field is highly relevant to understanding and achieving optimal nutrition because it allows us to personalize our diets based on individual genetic variations, thereby maximizing the health benefits we can derive from the food we eat. One of the fundamental principles of nutrigenomics is the concept of genetic variations, which refers to differences in the DNA sequence of individuals. These genetic variations can determine how our bodies respond to different nutrients, and can have significant implications for our overall health. For example, a particular genetic variant may increase an individual's risk of developing certain diseases, such as obesity or cardiovascular disease, in response to a specific diet. By studying these genetic variations and their interaction with nutrients, nutrigenomics seeks to identify the optimal diet that can minimize the risk of disease and promote optimal health for each individual. Another key aspect of nutrigenomics is the study of gene expression. Gene expression refers to the process by which the information coded in our genes is used to produce proteins, which are essential for the proper functioning of our cells and overall health. Nutrigenomics investigates how different dietary components can influence gene expression, either by turning genes on or off, or by modifying their activity levels.

For instance, certain nutrients, such as omega-3 fatty acids or vitamins, have been shown to modulate the expression of genes involved in inflammation or oxidative stress, which are known to contribute to the development of chronic diseases. By understanding how our dietary choices can influence gene expression, nutrigenomics allows us to optimize our diets to promote the expression of genes associated with health and well-being.

A major goal of nutrigenomics is to develop personalized nutrition strategies that take into account an individual's unique genetic makeup. Genetic testing allows individuals to identify specific genetic variations that may impact their nutrient metabolism or disease susceptibility. This genetic information can then be used to tailor dietary recommendations and interventions to each individual's specific needs. For example, an individual with a genetic variant that impairs their ability to metabolize a certain nutrient may need to adjust their diet or consider supplementation to ensure they are obtaining adequate amounts of that nutrient. By customizing dietary recommendations based on an individual's genetic profile, nutrigenomics can help optimize nutrition and promote optimal health outcomes.

The relevance of nutrigenomics to optimal nutrition lies in its potential to account for the wide variations in individuals' responses to diet and nutrition. It recognizes that one size does not fit all when it comes to nutrition, and that our genes play a crucial role in determining our nutritional needs. By understanding and utilizing the principles of nutrigenomics, we can personalize our diets to maximize the benefits we can derive from the foods we eat, and minimize our risk of developing diet-related diseases. This personalized approach to nutrition takes into account individual genetic variations, allowing us to tailor our diets to support our unique genetic makeup and promote optimal health. Nutrigenomics is a field that explores the intricate relationship between our genes and the food we consume. It investigates how genetic variations and dietary components can influence gene expression and cellular processes, with the goal of developing personalized nutrition strategies. This field is highly relevant to optimal nutrition, as it allows us to customize our diets based on individual genetic variations, optimizing nutrient metabolism and minimizing the risk of diet-related diseases. By understanding and harnessing the power of nutrigenomics, we can unlock the potential of optimal nutrition for holistic wellness.

GENETIC VARIATIONS CAN INFLUENCE AN INDIVIDUAL'S RESPONSE TO DIFFERENT FOODS

Genetic variations play a pivotal role in an individual's response to different foods, as they can greatly impact the way our bodies process and metabolize nutrients. The human genome is incredibly complex, with numerous genes involved in key processes such as digestion, nutrient absorption, and metabolism. These genes can contain different versions, or alleles, which can vary widely from person to person. The presence of certain alleles can confer advantages or disadvantages when it comes to processing specific nutrients, leading to differences in how individuals respond to different foods. One example of genetic variation affecting food response is the lactase gene, which is responsible for producing the enzyme lactase that breaks down lactose, the sugar found in milk and dairy products. Most mammals naturally lose the ability to digest lactose after infancy, as the production of lactase decreases. Some human populations have developed a genetic variation that allows them to continue producing lactase into adulthood, a trait known as lactase persistence. This genetic variation is more prevalent in populations that historically relied on dairying for sustenance, such as those of European descent. The ability to digest lactose in adulthood allows individuals with lactase persistence to comfortably consume dairy products, while those without this genetic variation may experience digestive symptoms such as bloating and diarrhea. Another example of genetic variation impacting food response is the gene that influences caffeine metabolism. This gene, known as CYP1A2, determines how quickly the body breaks down and eliminates caffeine. Individuals who possess a certain variant of this gene are classified as slow caffeine metabolizers, while those with another variant are fast caffeine metabolizers. Slow caffeine metabolizers take a longer time to process and eliminate caffeine from their bodies, leading to a heightened sensitivity to its effects. Fast caffeine metabolizers quickly metabolize and eliminate caffeine, which may require them to consume larger amounts of caffeine to feel the same effects. These genetic differences in caffeine metabolism can influence an individual's response to various caffeinated foods and beverages, such as coffee and tea. Genetic variations can also affect how our bodies respond to certain macronutrients, such as fats and carbohydrates. For instance, certain variations in genes involved in lipid metabolism have been shown to contribute to differences in cholesterol levels and response to dietary fat intake. Apolipoprotein E (APOE) is one such example, with different alleles influencing how efficiently the body processes and clears cholesterol from the bloodstream. Individuals with the APOE4 allele have been found to have a higher risk of elevated cholesterol levels and increased susceptibility to cardiovascular diseases when consuming a diet high in saturated fats. Individuals with the APOE2 allele may have a more efficient cholesterol metabolism, potentially leading to lower levels of circulating cholesterol even with a high-fat diet. This highlights the significance of genetic variations in lipid metabolism and their implications for an individual's response to dietary fats. Similarly, genetic variations can affect an individual's response to dietary carbohydrates. The gene known as TCF7L2 has been identified as a major player in determining an individual's risk of developing type 2 diabetes. Variants of this gene have been associated with differences in insulin secretion and insulin resistance, two key factors in the development of diabetes. Studies have shown that individuals with certain TCF7L2 variants have a higher risk of developing diabetes, especially when consuming a high-carbohydrate diet. These findings underscore how genetic variations can influence an individual's response to different sources of dietary carbohydrates, potentially impacting their long-term health outcomes.

Genetic variations can significantly impact an individual's response to different foods, ranging from lactose intolerance to caffeine sensitivity and the metabolism of fats and carbohydrates. Understanding these genetic variations can provide valuable insights into personalized nutrition and optimal health. By identifying individuals' unique genetic profiles, tailored dietary recommendations can be developed to promote better health outcomes and overall well-being. The study of genetic variations in food response opens up exciting possibilities for precision nutrition, where our diets can be optimized to suit our individual biological makeups for improved health and disease prevention.

NUTRIGENOMICS CAN HELP TAILOR NUTRITION PLANS FOR PERSONALIZED HEALTH

Nutrigenomics, the study of how our genes interact with the nutrients we consume, has gained considerable attention in recent years as a promising field in personalized nutrition. It takes into account the unique genetic makeup of individuals to tailor nutrition plans that optimize health outcomes. This approach recognizes that no two individuals are exactly alike, and that what works for one person may not work for another. By understanding how our genes influence our response to various nutrients, nutrigenomics aims to provide personalized nutrition recommendations that can prevent and manage chronic diseases.

One of the keyways nutrigenomics helps tailor nutrition plans for personalized health is by identifying genetic variations, known as single nucleotide polymorphisms (SNPs), that affect nutrient metabolism. These variations can impact how our bodies absorb, process, and utilize certain nutrients. For example, an individual with a particular SNP in the gene responsible for vitamin D metabolism may require higher vitamin D intake to maintain optimal levels in the body. By identifying these genetic variations through genetic testing, nutrigenomics can provide valuable information about an individual's specific nutrient needs and guide the development of personalized nutrition plans.

Nutrigenomics can help determine the ideal macronutrient ratios for individuals based on their genetic profiles. Macronutrients, including carbohydrates, proteins, and fats, make up the majority of our diet and play a crucial role in our overall health.

The optimal ratio of macronutrients may vary from person to person. By analyzing genetic variations related to macronutrient metabolism, nutrigenomics can provide insights into an individual's ability to process and utilize different macronutrients.

This information can guide the formulation of personalized nutrition plans that optimize macronutrient intake for optimal health outcomes. Nutrigenomics can inform dietary recommendations for individuals with specific genetic predispositions to certain health conditions. Genetic variations can influence an individual's risk of developing conditions such as obesity, diabetes, and cardiovascular disease. For example, certain SNPs may increase an individual's susceptibility to obesity by affecting their metabolism and appetite regulation. By identifying these genetic variations, nutrigenomics can help tailor nutrition plans that specifically address these genetic predispositions. This may involve recommending specific nutrients or dietary patterns that mitigate the risk of developing these conditions and promote overall wellness. Nutrigenomics can provide insights into how our genes influence our response to specific dietary factors, such as antioxidants, phytochemicals, and food allergens. Our ability to process and utilize these compounds varies among individuals due to genetic variations. For example, some individuals may have a genetic variation that affects their ability to metabolize certain antioxidants, reducing their potential health benefits. By identifying these genetic variations, nutrigenomics can help guide personalized nutrition plans that focus on maximizing the benefits of specific dietary factors for each individual.

Importantly, nutrigenomics also takes into account the dynamic nature of gene expression and the potential for genetic modifications through lifestyle interventions, such as diet and exercise.

Emerging research suggests that our lifestyle choices can influence gene expression and modify our genetic predispositions. This means that even individuals with a higher genetic risk for certain conditions can potentially mitigate their risk through targeted lifestyle interventions, including personalized nutrition plans. By integrating genetic information with lifestyle factors, nutrigenomics can help individuals understand how their genetic makeup interacts with their dietary choices and guide them towards effective strategies for personalized health.

Nutrigenomics holds great promise in tailoring nutrition plans for personalized health. By considering an individual's unique genetic makeup, nutrigenomics can identify genetic variations that affect nutrient metabolism, determine optimal macronutrient ratios, inform dietary recommendations for specific health conditions, and provide insights into the interaction between genes and dietary factors. This approach acknowledges the importance of individual differences in response to nutrition and aims to optimize health outcomes through personalized nutrition plans. As our understanding of the microbiome and genetic influences on health continues to grow, nutrigenomics will play a critical role in helping individuals achieve and maintain optimal health through targeted dietary interventions.

The field of microbiomics has gained significant attention in recent years, as researchers have discovered the profound impact that the microbiome has on human health. The microbiome refers to the diverse community of microorganisms that reside within our bodies, primarily in our digestive tract. These microorganisms, which include bacteria, viruses, fungi, and other microscopic organisms, play a crucial role in maintaining our overall health and well-being. Not only do they aid in the digestion and absorption of nutrients, but they also help to regulate our immune system and even influence our mental health.

Understanding the intricate relationship between the microbiome and human health is essential for developing strategies to optimize nutrition and promote holistic wellness.

One of the key factors that influence the composition and diversity of the microbiome is diet. The foods we consume provide the fuel and nourishment that these microorganisms need to thrive. Different types of dietary components, such as carbohydrates, proteins, and fats, can have varying effects on the microbiome. For example, a diet high in refined carbohydrates and sugars is associated with an imbalance in the microbiome, characterized by an overgrowth of certain bacteria that can contribute to inflammation and the development of chronic diseases. A diet rich in fiber, plant-based foods, and fermented foods can promote a healthy and diverse microbiome. Fiber serves as a prebiotic, a substance that nourishes beneficial bacteria in the gut. These bacteria ferment the fiber and produce short-chain fatty acids (SCFAs), which have anti-inflammatory properties and support gut health. Plant-based foods are rich in phytochemicals, which are bioactive compounds that have a positive impact on the microbiome. These compounds can modulate the composition of the microbiota and promote the growth of beneficial bacteria.

Fermented foods, such as yogurt, kefir, sauerkraut, and kimchi, are another important component of a gut-healthy diet. These foods are rich in probiotics, which are live microorganisms that confer health benefits when consumed in adequate amounts. Probiotics can help restore the balance of the microbiome and promote the growth of beneficial bacteria. In addition to their direct effect on the microbiome, probiotics can also enhance the immune system and improve digestive health.

A healthy and diverse microbiome is not only important for digestive health but also plays a vital role in immune function. The gut microbiota helps train the immune system to recognize harmless substances and respond appropriately to pathogens. When the microbiome is imbalanced, it can lead to immune dysregulation and an increased risk of infections and autoimmune diseases. Conversely, a healthy and diverse microbiome can enhance immune function and reduce the risk of chronic diseases. The impact of the microbiome extends beyond the digestive system and immune function. Emerging research suggests that the microbiome also has a significant influence on mental health. The gut-brain axis is a bidirectional communication system between the gut and the brain, which involves various pathways, including the immune system, the endocrine system, and the nervous system. The gut microbiota plays a crucial role in this communication, with emerging evidence linking alterations in the microbiome to conditions such as anxiety, depression, and neurodevelopmental disorders.

Considering the substantial impact that the microbiome has on human health, it is essential to adopt dietary strategies that support a healthy and diverse microbiome. Optimal nutrition involves consuming a balanced diet rich in nutrient-dense foods, such as fruits, vegetables, whole grains, lean proteins, and healthy fats. These foods provide the essential vitamins, minerals, and antioxidants needed for overall health and well-being.

It is crucial to prioritize fiber intake, as it serves as a prebiotic and supports the growth of beneficial bacteria in the gut. Including a variety of fiber-rich foods, such as fruits, vegetables, legumes, and whole grains, can ensure adequate fiber intake. Incorporating fermented foods into the diet, such as yogurt and sauerkraut, can provide probiotics that promote a healthy microbiome. The microbiome plays a critical role in human health and wellness. The foods we consume significantly influence the composition and diversity of the microbiome, which, in turn, affects our digestion, immune system, and even mental health. Adopting a diet that supports a healthy and diverse microbiome is essential for optimal nutrition and overall well-being. By incorporating fiber-rich foods and fermented foods into our diets, we can nourish our microbiomes and promote holistic wellness.

X. A HOLISTIC APPROACH TO OPTIMAL NUTRITION AND MICROBIOME HEALTH

The microbiome has gained increasing recognition for its critical role in human health and disease. Composed of trillions of microorganisms, including bacteria, fungi, viruses, and archaea, the microbiome constitutes a complex ecosystem that coexists in a symbiotic relationship with the human host. Recent research has shown that the composition of the microbiome plays a pivotal role in various physiological functions, such as digestion, metabolism, immune regulation, and even mental health. It is crucial to adopt a holistic approach to nutrition that considers the impact of diet on the microbiome, as this knowledge can potentially revolutionize our understanding of optimal nutrition and pave the way for personalized diet recommendations.

One of the key factors influencing the composition and diversity of the microbiome is the type and quality of food consumed. A diet rich in fibers and plant-based foods has been associated with a more diverse and stable microbiome, characterized by an abundance of beneficial bacteria. These beneficial bacteria produce short-chain fatty acids (SCFAs) through the fermentation of dietary fibers, which play a crucial role in maintaining gut health. SCFAs serve as an energy source for the cells lining the gut, promote the production of mucus, and regulate the immune response. a diet high in refined sugars, unhealthy fats, and processed foods has been shown to negatively impact the microbiome, leading to a decrease in diversity and an increase in harmful bacteria. This imbalance in the microbiome, known as dysbiosis, has been linked to various health conditions, including inflammatory bowel disease, obesity, and even mental disorders like depression and anxiety. Adopting a holistic approach to nutrition should go beyond focusing solely on macronutrients and calorie counting. Instead, it should encompass a more comprehensive understanding of the microbiome and its interactions with the food we eat. For example, prebiotics are a type of dietary fiber that cannot be digested by humans but serve as a fuel source for beneficial bacteria in the gut. By including prebiotic-rich foods, such as onions, garlic, and asparagus, in our diet, we can selectively promote the growth of beneficial bacteria, ultimately leading to a healthier microbiome. Similarly, probiotics, which are live microorganisms, can be beneficial in restoring and maintaining a balanced microbiome. Consuming fermented foods like yogurt, kefir, and sauerkraut can provide a variety of probiotic strains that can enhance gut health. A holistic approach to optimal nutrition also takes into account the impact of food processing and cooking methods on the microbiome. Processed foods often undergo high heat treatments and undergo extensive refinement processes that strip away essential nutrients and fiber. These foods, lacking in beneficial components, can promote dysbiosis and contribute to various health issues. Incorporating cooking methods that preserve the integrity of nutrients and minimize the destruction of beneficial bacteria, such as steaming or lightly sautéing vegetables, can maximize their nutritional value and support a healthy microbiome.

Importantly, a holistic approach to optimal nutrition should also consider the individuality of each person's microbiome. Recent advancements in microbiome research have revealed that each individual has a unique microbiome signature, shaped by a combination of genetic predispositions, early-life factors, and environmental influences, including diet. This personalized aspect of the microbiome underscores the need for individualized nutrition recommendations that cater to the specific needs of each person's microbiome. Future research should aim to unravel the complex interplay between the microbiome and various health conditions, allowing for the development of targeted interventions and personalized dietary strategies.

A holistic approach to optimal nutrition and microbiome health is crucial for maintaining overall wellness. By considering the impact of diet on the composition and diversity of the microbiome, we can make informed dietary choices that promote a balanced and thriving microbial community in our gut. A diet rich in fibers and plant-based foods, along with the inclusion of prebiotics and probiotics, serves as a foundation for supporting a healthy microbiome. Paying attention to food processing and cooking methods can further enhance the nutritional value of our meals. Recognizing the personalized nature of the microbiome emphasizes the need for individualized dietary recommendations to foster holistic wellness. Implementing these principles and understanding the science behind the microbiome can pave the way for a new era of optimal nutrition and microbiome-centered healthcare. Explanation of the importance of a holistic approach that considers both diet and lifestyle factors There has been a growing recognition of the importance of a holistic approach that considers both diet and lifestyle factors when it comes to optimal nutrition and overall wellness. The concept of holistic wellness emphasizes the interconnectedness of various aspects of health, recognizing that what we eat and how we live our lives can have a profound impact on our overall well-being. This approach is particularly relevant when it comes to understanding the role of the microbiome in human health.

The microbiome refers to the trillions of microorganisms that reside in and on our bodies, particularly in the gastrointestinal tract. These microorganisms, which include bacteria, viruses, and fungi, play a crucial role in various physiological processes and have a profound impact on our health. They aid in digestion, produce essential nutrients, regulate the immune system, and even influence our mood and behavior. In order to ensure the optimal functioning of our microbiomes, it is important to consider both diet and lifestyle factors.

Diet plays a critical role in shaping the composition and diversity of the microbiome. The foods we eat provide the nutrients and energy necessary for the growth and survival of the microorganisms in our gut. A diet rich in fiber, fruits, vegetables, and whole grains can promote the growth of beneficial bacteria in the gut, leading to a more diverse and balanced microbiome. A diet high in processed foods, sugar, and unhealthy fats can promote the growth of harmful bacteria and disrupt the delicate balance of the microbiome. One of the keyways in which diet influences the microbiome is through its impact on the production of short-chain fatty acids (SCFAs). SCFAs are a group of compounds that are produced by certain types of bacteria in the gut when they ferment dietary fiber. These compounds have been shown to have numerous health benefits, including improving gut health, reducing inflammation, and regulating metabolism. By consuming a diet high in dietary fiber, we can promote the production of SCFAs and support a healthy microbiome. In addition to diet, lifestyle factors also play a crucial role in shaping the microbiome. Stress, lack of sleep, and sedentary behavior can have a detrimental effect on the composition and diversity of the microbiome. Chronic stress, for example, has been shown to alter the balance of bacteria in the gut, leading to inflammation and impaired immune function. Similarly, inadequate sleep has been associated with alterations in the gut microbiome, including a decrease in microbial diversity.

Physical activity, on the other hand, has been shown to have a positive impact on the microbiome. Exercise has been found to increase the abundance of beneficial bacteria in the gut, reduce inflammation, and improve metabolic health. Regular exercise can also enhance the diversity of the microbiome, which is considered a marker of a healthy gut. By taking a holistic approach that considers both diet and lifestyle factors, we can optimize our nutrition and promote the health of our microbiomes. This means not only focusing on the types of foods we eat but also considering how our daily habits and routines can influence our gut health. It involves finding a balance between nutritious, whole foods and incorporating regular physical activity, managing stress levels, and getting adequate sleep.

A holistic approach that considers both diet and lifestyle factors is crucial for optimal nutrition and overall wellness. By recognizing the importance of the microbiome and its impact on human health, we can make informed choices about what we eat and how we live our lives. This involves consuming a diet rich in fiber and whole foods, incorporating regular exercise, managing stress levels, and getting adequate sleep. By prioritizing these aspects of our lives, we can support a healthy microbiome and improve our overall health and well-being.

THE ROLE OF PHYSICAL ACTIVITY, STRESS MANAGEMENT, AND SLEEP IN MICROBIOME HEALTH

In addition to optimal nutrition, other lifestyle factors also play a crucial role in maintaining a healthy microbiome. Physical activity, stress management, and sleep are three important components that significantly impact the composition and function of our microbiota. Regular physical activity has been associated with numerous health benefits, including the promotion of a diverse and robust microbiome. Exercise has been shown to increase the abundance of beneficial bacteria, such as those belonging to the phyla Bacteroidetes, Firmicutes, and Actinobacteria. These bacteria are involved in the production of short-chain fatty acids (SCFAs), which have anti-inflammatory properties and help to maintain gut barrier integrity. Physical activity has been demonstrated to reduce the abundance of potentially harmful bacteria such as pathogenic Proteobacteria. The mechanisms through which exercise influences the microbiome are not yet fully understood, but it is believed that changes in gut motility, immune function, and systemic inflammation play a role. Engaging in regular physical activity not only benefits our overall health but also contributes to a healthier gut microbiome. Stress, a common feature of modern life, has been shown to have a significant impact on the gut microbiome. Chronic stress has been associated with alterations in the composition of the microbiota, leading to dysbiosis and increased susceptibility to various diseases. Stress activates the hypothalamic-pituitary-adrenal (HPA) axis, leading to the release of stress hormones such as cortisol. These hormones have been shown to directly impact the gut microbial community by altering gut permeability, modulating immune function, and affecting the production of SCFAs. Stress-induced changes in eating behavior, such as increased consumption of highly processed foods and altered food preferences, can further impact the diversity and composition of the microbiome. Effective stress management strategies are essential for maintaining a healthy microbiome. Techniques such as Mindfulness meditation, yoga, deep breathing exercises, and engaging in hobbies or activities that promote relaxation can help to reduce stress levels and promote a healthy gut microbiome. Sleep is another critical factor that influences the health of our microbiota. Disruptions in sleep patterns, such as inadequate sleep duration or poor sleep quality, have been associated with alterations in the gut microbiome. Sleep deprivation has been shown to decrease the abundance of beneficial bacteria such as Bacteroidetes and increase the abundance of potentially harmful bacteria such as Firmicutes. These changes in microbial composition have been linked to increased inflammation, impaired gut barrier function, and metabolic disorders. Sleep disturbances have also been shown to disrupt the circadian rhythm, which is known to play a crucial role in maintaining a healthy gut microbiome. The circadian rhythm regulates various physiological processes, including the production and secretion of digestive enzymes, the motility of the gastrointestinal tract, and the turnover of intestinal epithelial cells. Disruptions in the circadian rhythm can lead to dysbiosis and increased susceptibility to gut-related diseases. Prioritizing adequate and quality sleep is essential for supporting a healthy microbiome. Physical activity, stress management, and sleep are important factors that influence the health and diversity of our microbiome. Regular exercise promotes the growth of beneficial bacteria and reduces the abundance of potentially harmful bacteria. Effective stress management strategies help to maintain a diverse and balanced microbiota by minimizing the negative impact of stress on the gut microbial community. Adequate sleep duration and quality support a healthy microbiome by ensuring the proper functioning of physiological processes regulated by the circadian rhythm. By incorporating these lifestyle factors into our daily routine, we can optimize our microbiome health and promote overall well-being.

ADDITIONAL FACTORS, SUCH AS ENVIRONMENTAL EXPOSURES, THAT MAY IMPACT THE MICROBIOME

In addition to diet and lifestyle factors, environmental exposures can also play a significant role in shaping the microbiome. The environment in which we live is filled with various microorganisms that can potentially impact our microbial communities. For example, exposure to different types of bacteria, viruses, fungi, and other microorganisms can influence the composition and diversity of our microbiome. Research has shown that individuals living in urban areas have a different microbiome compared to those living in rural areas. This difference may be partly due to the higher levels of pollution and other environmental contaminants in urban settings. Pollutants such as particulate matter, heavy metals, and pesticides have been shown to disrupt the balance of the microbiome and have potential adverse effects on human health. Air pollution, in particular, has received considerable attention in recent years for its impact on the microbiome. Studies have demonstrated that exposure to air pollutants, such as nitrogen dioxide and particulate matter, can alter the composition of the gut microbiome. These pollutants can induce changes in the abundance of certain bacterial species and affect the overall diversity of the microbiome. Air pollution has been associated with an increased risk of various health conditions, including respiratory diseases, cardiovascular diseases, and metabolic disorders. It is theorized that the disruption of the microbiome could be one of the mechanisms through which air pollution exerts its detrimental effects on health. Another important environmental factor that can influence the microbiome is the use of antibiotics. Antibiotics are commonly prescribed medications that are effective in treating bacterial infections. They can also have unintended consequences on the microbiome. Antibiotics work by killing or inhibiting the growth of bacteria, and they do not discriminate between harmful bacteria and beneficial bacteria in the gut. As a result, antibiotic use can disrupt the balance of the microbiome, leading to a decrease in microbial diversity and an overgrowth of opportunistic pathogens. This disruption can have long-term consequences on health, as a healthy microbiome is important for various physiological processes, such as digestion, immune response, and nutrient metabolism. The excessive use of antibiotics is particularly concerning as it can lead to the emergence of antibiotic-resistant bacteria. These bacteria have acquired genetic mutations or acquired resistance genes that allow them to survive the effects of antibiotics. The overuse and misuse of antibiotics in both humans and animals have contributed to the spread of antibiotic-resistant bacteria, posing a significant public health challenge. In addition to directly impacting human health, these antibiotic-resistant bacteria can also indirectly affect the microbiome by transferring their resistance genes to other bacteria in the gut. This can further disrupt the composition and function of the microbiome and make it more susceptible to infections. Other environmental exposures, such as exposure to chemicals and toxins, can also impact the microbiome. For instance, certain chemicals found in personal care products, cleaning agents, and pesticides have been shown to have antimicrobial properties. Exposure to these chemicals can disrupt the delicate balance of the microbiome and potentially contribute to the development of various health conditions. Certain toxins produced by harmful algal blooms and environmental pollutants can exert toxic effects on the gut microbiome. These toxins can damage the intestinal lining and disrupt the communication between the gut microbiota and the host, leading to inflammation and other adverse health effects.

The microbiome is not solely influenced by diet and lifestyle factors, but also by various environmental exposures. Air pollution, antibiotic use, and exposure to chemicals and toxins can all impact the composition and diversity of the microbiome. These factors have the potential to disrupt the delicate balance of the microbiome and contribute to the development of various health conditions. Understanding the role of these environmental exposures in shaping the microbiome is crucial for developing strategies to maintain a healthy microbiome and promote overall wellness. The human microbiome is a complex and vast ecosystem that consists of trillions of microorganisms, including bacteria, viruses, and fungi, residing in and on our bodies. This intricate microbial community plays a crucial role in maintaining our health and well-being. Recent advancements in research have shed light on the significant impact of the microbiome on various aspects of human physiology, including digestion, metabolism, and even mental health. Understanding the microbial composition and function in our bodies can pave the way for optimizing our nutrition and improving our overall health.

One of the fundamental ways in which the microbiome influences our health is through its involvement in digestion and metabolism. Our gut microbiome, in particular, plays a pivotal role in breaking down and extracting nutrients from the food we consume. The microbes residing in our gastrointestinal tract possess a diverse array of enzymes that help break down complex carbohydrates, proteins, and fats that our own digestive enzymes cannot fully process. Through this symbiotic relationship, our gut microbiome helps us extract additional energy and nutrients from our diet, improving our overall nutrient absorption. The microbiome also has a profound impact on our metabolism. Recent studies have shown that the composition of our gut microbiota can influence our energy expenditure and the way we metabolize certain nutrients, such as carbohydrates and fats. Imbalances or disruptions in the gut microbiota, known as dysbiosis, have been linked to conditions such as obesity and metabolic disorders. For instance, individuals with a higher abundance of certain bacteria in their gut, such as Firmicutes, may have a tendency to extract more energy from their food, leading to weight gain and increased risk of obesity.

In addition to its role in digestion and metabolism, the microbiome also affects our immune system and overall immune health. The gut microbiota, in particular, plays a crucial role in training and modulating our immune system. The interaction between the microbes in our gut and the cells of our immune system helps shape our immune response and tolerance to both harmless and harmful substances. This complex interplay is essential for maintaining immune homeostasis and protecting against infections and inflammatory diseases.

Research has begun to uncover the important relationship between the gut microbiome and mental health. The gut-brain axis, a bidirectional communication network connecting the gut and the central nervous system, has been shown to be influenced by the microbiome. Studies have found that alterations in the gut microbiota composition and function can contribute to the development of mental health disorders, such as anxiety and depression. For instance, certain strains of bacteria, such as Lactobacillus and Bifidobacterium, have been found to produce neurotransmitters and other metabolites that can influence brain function and mood. Given the significant impact of the microbiome on our health, it is important to consider how our dietary choices can influence this complex ecosystem. Our diet directly impacts the composition and function of the microbiome. Certain dietary components, such as fiber, act as prebiotics, providing fuel for beneficial bacteria in the gut. Fermentable fibers, found in plant-based foods like fruits, vegetables, and whole grains, are especially important for supporting a diverse and healthy gut microbiota. Diets high in processed foods and saturated fats have been associated with dysbiosis and a less favorable microbial composition. The Western diet, characterized by its high sugar and fat content, has been found to promote the growth of harmful bacteria and reduce the abundance of beneficial microbes. This dysbiosis can contribute to chronic inflammation, insulin resistance, and increased risk of metabolic disorders. Adopting a diet that supports a diverse and balanced microbiome, such as a plant-based diet rich in fiber and fermented foods, can be beneficial for both our gut health and overall well-being. The microbiome is a fascinating and intricate ecosystem that influences various aspects of our health. From digestion and metabolism to immune function and mental health, the microbiome is a key player in maintaining our overall well-being. Understanding the role of the microbiome in human health allows us to make informed dietary choices that can op-

timize our nutrition and promote holistic wellness.
By nourishing our microbiome with a diverse and healthy diet, we can support a thriving microbial community that works in harmony with our bodies for improved health and vitality.

XI. STRATEGIES FOR IMPROVING THE MICROBIOME THROUGH NUTRITION

One of the most effective strategies for improving the microbiome through nutrition is to consume a diverse range of plant-based foods. Research has shown that a high-fiber diet, rich in fruits, vegetables, whole grains, and legumes, can lead to a greater diversity of gut bacteria. This is because these foods are rich in prebiotics, which are indigestible fibers that serve as food for beneficial gut bacteria. By providing these bacteria with the nutrients they need to thrive, a high-fiber diet can promote a healthy and balanced microbiome. In addition to consuming a diverse range of plant-based foods, it is also important to limit the consumption of refined sugars and processed foods. These types of foods have been shown to promote the growth of harmful bacteria in the gut, which can disrupt the balance of the microbiome. By reducing the intake of these foods and focusing on whole, unprocessed foods, individuals can support the growth of beneficial bacteria and improve their overall gut health. Another strategy for improving the microbiome through nutrition is to include fermented foods in the diet. Fermented foods, such as yogurt, sauerkraut, and kimchi, contain live bacteria that can colonize the gut and provide additional benefits to the microbiome. These foods are especially rich in probiotics, which are live microorganisms that confer health benefits to the host when consumed in adequate amounts. Probiotics have been shown to improve digestion, strengthen the immune system, and reduce inflammation in the gut. By incorporating fermented foods into their diet, individuals can introduce these beneficial bacteria into their gut and support a healthy and diverse microbiome. In addition to consuming a diverse range of plant-based foods and fermented foods, it is also important to consider the role of macronutrients in microbiome health. Research has shown that the composition of the diet, particularly the ratio of carbohydrates to fats to proteins, can have a significant impact on the microbiome. A diet high in fat and low in fiber, for example, has been shown to promote the growth of harmful bacteria in the gut, while a diet high in fiber and low in fat promotes the growth of beneficial bacteria. By focusing on a balanced diet that includes adequate amounts of each macronutrient, individuals can support the growth of beneficial bacteria and maintain a healthy microbiome. The timing of meals and the frequency of eating can also influence the microbiome. Research has shown that intermittent fasting, or periods of extended fasting followed by periods of eating, can have a positive impact on gut health. Intermittent fasting has been shown to increase the diversity of gut bacteria, improve insulin sensitivity, and reduce inflammation in the gut. By incorporating intermittent fasting into their routine, individuals can support the growth of beneficial bacteria and improve their overall gut health. It is important to consider the role of lifestyle factors, such as stress and physical activity, in microbiome health. Chronic stress has been shown to alter the composition of the microbiome, leading to an imbalance of bacteria in the gut. Conversely, regular physical activity has been shown to promote the growth of beneficial bacteria and improve gut health. By managing stress levels and engaging in regular physical activity, individuals can support the growth of beneficial bacteria and improve their overall microbiome health. Improving the microbiome through nutrition is a complex process that requires a multi-faceted approach. Consuming a diverse range of plant-based foods, limiting the intake of refined sugars and processed foods, incorporating fermented foods into the diet, and considering the role of macronutrients, meal timing, and lifestyle factors are all strategies that can support a healthy and balanced microbiome. By understanding the impact of nutrition on the microbiome and adopting these strategies, individuals can improve their gut health and promote holistic wellness.

PRACTICAL STEPS INDIVIDUALS CAN TAKE TO IMPROVE THEIR MICROBIOME THROUGH NUTRITION

The microbiome, which refers to the diverse community of microorganisms that inhabit the human body, has a profound impact on our health and well-being. Research has shown that the composition of our microbiome is heavily influenced by our diet, and by making certain dietary choices, we can work towards improving our microbiome and promoting better overall health. One practical step individuals can take to improve their microbiome through nutrition is to increase their consumption of fiber-rich foods. Fiber serves as a source of nourishment for beneficial bacteria in the gut, known as probiotics, allowing them to thrive and multiply. Foods such as whole grains, legumes, fruits, and vegetables are excellent sources of fiber. Including a variety of these fiber-rich foods in one's diet can help support the growth of a diverse and healthy microbiome. Consuming foods that are rich in polyphenols, which are compounds found in certain fruits, vegetables, and nuts, can also promote the growth of beneficial bacteria in the gut. Polyphenols have been shown to have prebiotic-like effects, meaning they can selectively stimulate the growth of specific beneficial bacteria. Foods such as berries, cherries, broccoli, and green tea are particularly rich in polyphenols and can be incorporated into one's diet to support a healthier microbiome. Another practical step individuals can take is to consume fermented foods. Fermented foods, such as yogurt, sauerkraut, kimchi, and kefir, contain live bacteria that can colonize the gut and positively influence the composition of the microbiome. These live bacteria, known as probiotics, can help restore and maintain a healthy balance of gut bacteria. Including a serving of fermented foods in one's daily diet is a simple and effective way to improve the microbiome. In addition to incorporating specific foods, individuals can also improve their microbiome by avoiding certain dietary factors that can negatively impact the balance of gut bacteria. One important factor is the excessive consumption of processed foods high in sugar and unhealthy fats. These foods have been shown to alter the composition of the microbiome, favoring the growth of harmful bacteria and leading to inflammation and other detrimental effects on health. By reducing the intake of these processed foods and instead opting for whole, unprocessed foods, individuals can help maintain a healthier balance of gut bacteria. Another factor to consider is the use of antibiotics. While antibiotics can be essential for treating bacterial infections, they can also disrupt the delicate balance of the microbiome by killing off both harmful and beneficial bacteria. Whenever possible, individuals should work with their healthcare provider to minimize unnecessary antibiotic use and explore alternative treatments. Managing stress levels is crucial for maintaining a healthy microbiome. Chronic stress has been shown to have negative effects on the microbiome, leading to changes in gut bacteria composition and increased risk of various health conditions. Engaging in stress-reducing activities, such as regular exercise, mindful practices like meditation or deep breathing, and getting enough sleep, can help support a healthier microbiome. Improving one's microbiome through nutrition requires a multi-faceted approach. By increasing the consumption of fiber-rich foods, incorporating polyphenol-rich foods, consuming fermented foods, avoiding processed foods and unnecessary antibiotics, and managing stress levels, individuals can take practical steps towards enhancing their gut health. Embracing these dietary habits can help promote a diverse and beneficial microbiome, leading to improved overall health and well-being.

HOW TO INCORPORATE MORE WHOLE, UNPROCESSED FOODS INTO THE DIET

Incorporating more whole, unprocessed foods into our diet is essential for achieving optimal nutrition and improving our overall health. Whole foods, such as fruits, vegetables, whole grains, and lean proteins, provide a rich array of nutrients, fiber, and bioactive compounds that are vital for our well-being. By consuming these foods in their natural state, we can maximize their nutritional benefits while minimizing the intake of added sugars, unhealthy fats, and artificial ingredients commonly found in processed foods. To successfully integrate more whole, unprocessed foods into our diet, we should focus on meal planning, mindful eating, and exploring new recipes and food combinations. One effective strategy for incorporating more whole, unprocessed foods into our diet is meal planning. Planning our meals in advance allows us to make intentional choices and ensures that we have the necessary ingredients on hand. This practice can help us avoid relying on convenience foods or take-out meals, which are often highly processed and lacking in nutrients. By dedicating a specific time each week to plan our meals, we can design a menu that includes a variety of whole foods, ensuring that we obtain a wide range of nutrients and flavors. Meal planning can help us save time and money by reducing food waste and making the most of our grocery shopping trips. Mindful eating is another important aspect of incorporating whole, unprocessed foods into our diet. By practicing Mindfulness while eating, we can cultivate a deeper awareness of our body's hunger and fullness cues, as well as our cravings and emotional triggers. This heightened awareness can help us make conscious choices about the foods we consume and the portions we serve ourselves. By savoring each bite and paying attention to the flavors, textures, and aromas of our meals, we can develop a greater appreciation for whole, unprocessed foods and the nourishment they provide.

Exploring new recipes and food combinations is also crucial for incorporating more whole, unprocessed foods into our diet. Many individuals may feel overwhelmed or uninspired when it comes to cooking with these types of ingredients. With a little creativity and experimentation, we can discover a whole new world of flavors and textures that will make us look forward to each meal. Trying out different cooking methods, such as roasting, steaming, or grilling, can enhance the natural flavors of whole foods. Experimenting with herbs, spices, and homemade dressings can add complexity and depth to our dishes without relying on processed sauces or seasonings. By expanding our culinary repertoire and finding joy in the kitchen, we can easily incorporate more whole, unprocessed foods into our daily meals. Incorporating more whole, unprocessed foods into our diet is not only beneficial for our individual health but also for our entire community and the environment. Whole foods are often locally sourced, supporting local farmers and reducing our carbon footprint. By choosing whole foods over processed counterparts, we can help decrease the demand for industrial agriculture, which is harmful to ecosystems and contributes to greenhouse gas emissions. Consuming whole, unprocessed foods can promote sustainable eating habits, as they often require less packaging and processing, reducing waste.

Incorporating more whole, unprocessed foods into our diet is a crucial step towards achieving optimal nutrition and improving our overall health. By meal planning, practicing mindful eating, and exploring new recipes and food combinations, we can easily integrate these nutritious foods into our daily meals. Not only will we reap the benefits of their rich array of nutrients and bio-active compounds, but we will also contribute to a more sustainable and environmentally-friendly food system. Making the conscious choice to prioritize whole, unprocessed foods is a powerful way to fuel our bodies, nurture our microbiomes, and promote holistic wellness.

RESOURCES AND TOOLS FOR INDIVIDUALS TO TRACK AND MONITOR THEIR MICROBIOME HEALTH

There has been a growing interest in understanding the role of the microbiome in human health. As we delve deeper into the fascinating world of our gut bacteria, scientists have developed various resources and tools to help individuals track and monitor their microbiome health. These resources and tools aim to provide valuable insights into the composition and function of our gut microbiota, enabling us to make informed decisions regarding our diet and lifestyle. One such resource is the advent of microbiome testing kits, which allow individuals to obtain a detailed analysis of the bacteria present in their gut. These kits typically involve the collection of a stool sample, which is then sent to a laboratory for analysis. The lab utilizes advanced sequencing techniques to identify the different types of bacteria in the sample and provides a comprehensive report detailing the abundance of specific microbial species. This information can help individuals understand the composition of their microbiome and make personalized dietary choices that promote a healthy and diverse gut microbiota. There are various online platforms and databases that serve as valuable resources for individuals looking to explore the world of the microbiome. One such platform is the American Gut Project, which is a crowdsourced research initiative aimed at understanding the gut microbiome's diversity and its impact on human health. Participants in the project can contribute their own microbiome data and gain access to a wealth of information about the microbiome. This platform not only allows individuals to monitor their own microbiome health but also contributes to the collective knowledge of the scientific community about the microbiome.

Another resource that individuals can utilize to track their microbiome health is the development of smartphone applications specifically designed for this purpose. These applications use algorithms and machine learning technology to analyze data from multiple sources, such as dietary intake, exercise habits, and symptoms, to provide personalized recommendations for improving gut health. By tracking various lifestyle factors and their impact on the gut microbiota, these applications help individuals make informed decisions regarding their diet and lifestyle choices. Some applications even allow for real-time monitoring of the microbiome, providing individuals with instant feedback on the effect of their activities on their gut bacteria.

In addition to these resources, there are various research initiatives and studies that individuals can participate in to monitor their microbiome health. These studies often provide participants with microbiome testing kits and detailed reports on their gut bacteria composition. By participating in such studies, individuals not only gain insights into their own microbiome health but also contribute to the advancement of scientific knowledge in the field. There are online communities and forums dedicated to discussing and sharing information about the microbiome. These platforms provide a space for individuals to ask questions, share experiences, and learn from others who are also interested in optimizing their gut health. These communities often include experts in the field who can provide guidance and help individuals interpret their microbiome data.

The growing interest in the microbiome has led to the development of various resources and tools that individuals can utilize to track and monitor their microbiome health. Microbiome testing kits, online platforms, smartphone applications, research initiatives, and online communities are all valuable resources that provide individuals with insights into their gut bacterial composition, allowing them to make informed decisions regarding their diet and lifestyle choices. As we continue to uncover the complex relationship between the microbiome and human health, these resources and tools will likely play an increasingly important role in promoting holistic wellness through optimal nutrition. There has been a growing interest in the science of the microbiome and its impact on human health. The microbiome refers to the community of microorganisms that live in and on our bodies, including bacteria, viruses, fungi, and other microbes. These microbes have been found to play a crucial role in our overall well-being, influencing everything from digestion to immunity. Understanding the microbiome and its relationship to nutrition can lead to profound insights into how we can optimize our health. One of the keyways that nutrition influences the microbiome is through the foods we eat. Our diet has a direct impact on the composition and diversity of our microbiome. Certain foods can promote the growth of beneficial bacteria, while others can lead to an overgrowth of harmful bacteria. For example, a diet high in fiber has been shown to increase the abundance of beneficial bacteria in the gut. Fiber acts as a prebiotic, providing nourishment for these bacteria and helping them thrive. A diet high in processed foods and sugar can disrupt the balance of bacteria in the gut, leading to dysbiosis, or an imbalance of microbial communities. This dysbiosis has been associated with a range of health issues, including obesity, diabetes, and inflammatory bowel disease.

In addition to influencing the composition of the microbiome, nutrition can also affect the function of these microorganisms. The microbiome is involved in a wide range of physiological processes, including digestion, immune function, and even mental health. Nutrition can modulate these functions by influencing the activity of the microbiome. For example, certain nutrients have been found to promote the production of short-chain fatty acids (SCFAs) by the microbiome. SCFAs are important signaling molecules that play a role in regulating immune function and inflammation. A diet rich in plant-based foods, such as fruits, vegetables, and whole grains, has been shown to increase the production of SCFAs and promote a healthy inflammatory response. Conversely, a diet high in saturated fats and processed foods can lead to the production of harmful metabolites by the microbiome, contributing to chronic inflammation and other health problems. Understanding the relationship between nutrition and the microbiome can also help us personalize dietary recommendations for individuals. The composition and function of the microbiome can vary widely among individuals, depending on factors such as genetics, age, and environmental exposures. By analyzing the microbiome, scientists can identify specific microbial signatures associated with health or disease. This information can then be used to develop personalized dietary recommendations that target the individual's unique microbiome. For example, someone with a low abundance of certain beneficial bacteria may benefit from consuming foods that promote their growth, such as fermented foods or probiotic supplements. Someone with an overgrowth of harmful bacteria may need to avoid certain foods that fuel their growth, such as sugary beverages or processed meats. By tailoring dietary recommendations to the individual's microbiome, we can optimize their health and well-being. The science of the microbiome has provided valuable insights into the relationship between nutrition and human health. Our diet plays a significant role in shaping the composition and function of the microbiome, which in turn influences a wide range of physiological processes. Understanding this intricate web of interactions can help us develop optimal nutrition strategies that promote a healthy microbiome and improve our overall well-being. By choosing the right foods and nutrients, we can nourish our microbial communities and unlock the potential for greater holistic wellness. The microbiome is a fascinating frontier in health research, and continued exploration of its impact on human health will undoubtedly lead to new discoveries and better strategies for disease prevention and treatment.

XII. CASE STUDIES: SUCCESS STORIES OF MICROBIOME-DRIVEN NUTRITION

There have been numerous case studies documenting the success of microbiome-driven nutrition in improving the health of individuals. These success stories serve as evidence of the profound impact that the microbiome can have on our overall well-being. One such example is the case of Sarah, a 35-year-old woman who had been struggling with digestive issues for years. Sarah had tried various diets and medications, but nothing seemed to alleviate her symptoms. After consulting with a nutritionist who focused on microbiome-driven nutrition, Sarah began to see significant improvements in her health.

The nutritionist first conducted a comprehensive analysis of Sarah's microbiome through stool testing. This analysis revealed an imbalance in Sarah's gut bacteria, with an overgrowth of harmful bacteria and a deficiency of beneficial bacteria. Armed with this information, the nutritionist designed a personalized diet plan for Sarah to restore balance to her microbiome. The plan included a variety of fermented foods, such as yogurt, sauerkraut, and kefir, which are rich in probiotics that promote the growth of beneficial bacteria in the gut.

Within a few weeks of following the diet plan, Sarah began to notice a dramatic improvement in her digestion. Her bloating and abdominal pain decreased, and her bowel movements became regular and less uncomfortable. Sarah also experienced a boost in her energy levels and overall mood. Encouraged by these positive changes, Sarah continued to adhere to the microbiome-driven diet and saw further improvements in her health over time. Her skin cleared up, she lost excess weight, and her immune system seemed stronger than ever.

Another inspiring success story is that of Mark, a 50-year-old man who had been struggling with chronic inflammation for years. Mark suffered from joint pain, stiffness, and frequent infections, which greatly affected his quality of life. Despite trying various anti-inflammatory medications, Mark found little relief. Desperate for a solution, Mark turned to microbiome-driven nutrition as a last resort. Upon analyzing Mark's microbiome, it was discovered that he had a high level of inflammation-promoting bacteria in his gut. Armed with this knowledge, Mark's nutritionist tailored a diet plan that focused on reducing inflammation and promoting a healthy balance of gut bacteria. This included foods rich in anti-inflammatory compounds, such as fatty fish, olive oil, and leafy greens. The plan also emphasized the consumption of prebiotic-rich foods, such as onions, garlic, and asparagus, to nourish the growth of beneficial bacteria. To Mark's surprise, he began to see significant improvements in his symptoms within just a few weeks of starting the diet plan. His joint pain diminished, and he experienced greater flexibility and mobility. Mark also noticed that he was falling ill less frequently and recovering more quickly when he did. Over time, Mark's inflammation markers decreased, further confirming the positive impact of microbiome-driven nutrition on his health. These case studies demonstrate the power of microbiome-driven nutrition in addressing specific health concerns. By understanding the unique composition of each individual's microbiome, nutritionists can develop personalized diet plans that target the root causes of various conditions. Rather than simply treating the symptoms, these diet plans focus on restoring balance and promoting the growth of beneficial bacteria.

The success stories of Sarah and Mark provide hope and inspiration for those who have struggled with chronic health issues. They serve as a reminder that optimal nutrition plays a crucial role in maintaining a healthy microbiome and overall well-being. By harnessing the power of the microbiome through personalized diet plans, individuals can take control of their health and unlock their body's natural ability to heal and thrive.

Presentation of real-life examples of individuals who have transformed their health through microbiome-focused nutrition Presentation of real-life examples of individuals who have transformed their health through microbiome-focused nutrition can serve as powerful motivators for people seeking to improve their own well-being. Through the adoption of specific dietary changes aimed at nurturing a healthy microbiome, these individuals have experienced remarkable transformations in their overall health and well-being. One such example is that of Sarah, a 35-year-old woman who had struggled with chronic digestive issues for years. Despite visiting numerous doctors and trying various medications, Sarah found no relief from her symptoms. Frustrated and desperate, she began researching alternative approaches to her condition and came across the concept of microbiome-focused nutrition. Sarah decided to overhaul her diet, eliminating processed foods and incorporating more fiber-rich plant-based foods. Within a few months, Sarah noticed a significant improvement in her digestion, with less bloating and discomfort. She experienced an unexpected side effect – her mood improved, and she felt more energized throughout the day. Inspired by her own positive experiences, Sarah decided to pursue further education in the field of nutrition to help others achieve similar transformations.

Another individual whose health was transformed by microbiome-focused nutrition is Mike, a 43-year-old man who had struggled with obesity for most of his adult life. Being overweight not only affected Mike's self-esteem but also put him at risk for various obesity-related diseases. Determined to make a change, Mike sought the help of a registered dietitian who introduced him to the concept of the microbiome and its influence on weight management. Mike began incorporating more fiber-rich foods, such as fruits, vegetables, and whole grains, into his diet while reducing his intake of processed and sugary foods.

Over time, he noticed significant weight loss and improvements in his overall health. Not only did his digestion improve, but his blood pressure and cholesterol levels also normalized. Mike experienced increased energy levels and found that he no longer relied on unhealthy, sugary snacks for a mid-afternoon pick-me-up. Today, Mike serves as a source of inspiration for others struggling with weight management, sharing his personal journey and the positive impact that microbiome-focused nutrition had on his well-being. These real-life examples demonstrate the profound impact that microbiome-focused nutrition can have on an individual's health. By understanding how the foods we eat influence our microbiomes, we can make informed choices that promote a thriving microbial community. This, in turn, can lead to improvements in various aspects of our well-being, ranging from digestion to mood and overall vitality.

These examples underline the importance of personalized approaches to nutrition, as what works for one person may not work for another. Sarah's experience with plant-based nutrition highlights the power of incorporating fiber-rich foods into one's diet, while Mike's success with weight management emphasizes the significance of reducing processed and sugary foods.

The presentation of real-life examples of individuals who have transformed their health through microbiome-focused nutrition serves as a valuable source of inspiration and motivation for those looking to improve their own well-being. Sarah and Mike's experiences demonstrate the transformative power of adopting dietary changes aimed at nurturing a healthy microbiome. From improved digestion to weight loss and increased energy, these individuals experienced a wide range of health benefits as a result of their nutrition-focused interventions. These examples highlight the importance of understanding the microbiome and its impact on human health, as well as the need for personalized approaches to nutrition. By harnessing the science of the microbiome, individuals can optimize their nutrition for holistic wellness, unlocking their full potential for health and vitality.

THE SPECIFIC CHANGES THEY MADE TO THEIR DIET AND LIFESTYLE

In order to optimize their microbiome and overall health, many individuals have chosen to make specific changes to their diet and lifestyle. One of the most common changes is a shift towards a more plant-based diet. By increasing their intake of fruits, vegetables, whole grains, and legumes, individuals are able to introduce a wide variety of beneficial bacteria into their gut. These plant-based foods are rich in prebiotics, which serve as food for the healthy bacteria in the gut, promoting their growth and diversity. A plant-based diet is typically lower in fat and higher in fiber, both of which are key factors in maintaining a healthy gut microbiome. Another specific change that individuals have made to their diet is the introduction of fermented foods. Fermented foods such as yogurt, sauerkraut, and kimchi are rich sources of probiotics, which are live bacteria that have been shown to have numerous health benefits. These probiotics can help to strengthen the gut barrier, enhance immune function, and reduce inflammation. By incorporating fermented foods into their diet, individuals are able to introduce these beneficial bacteria into their gut, promoting a healthier microbiome. In addition to changes in diet, individuals have also made specific lifestyle changes to optimize their microbiome. One change is the reduction in the use of antibiotics. While antibiotics can be life-saving in certain situations, they can also have a detrimental effect on the gut microbiome. Antibiotics work by killing off both harmful and beneficial bacteria, leading to an imbalance in the gut. This imbalance, known as dysbiosis, can have a negative impact on health. By being more judicious in their use of antibiotics and exploring alternative treatments when appropriate, individuals are able to minimize the disruption to their microbiome. Another lifestyle change individuals have made is the reduction in stress levels. Chronic stress has been shown to have a negative impact on the gut microbiome, leading to a decrease in beneficial bacteria and an increase in harmful bacteria. This imbalance in the microbiome can contribute to a variety of health issues, including digestive disorders, immune dysfunction, and mental health disorders. To combat this, individuals have embraced stress-reducing activities such as yoga, meditation, and regular exercise. These activities have been shown to not only reduce stress, but also positively influence the gut microbiome by promoting the growth of beneficial bacteria. Individuals have also focused on improving their sleep habits to optimize their microbiome. Sleep deprivation has been linked to an imbalance in the gut microbiota, with a decrease in beneficial bacteria and an increase in harmful bacteria. Disruptions in sleep can lead to increased inflammation in the body, which can further negatively impact the gut microbiome. By prioritizing sleep and adopting healthy sleep habits, individuals are able to promote a healthier microbiome and overall well-being. Individuals have made specific changes to their hygiene routines to optimize their microbiome. While hygiene is important for preventing the spread of harmful pathogens, excessive cleanliness can also disrupt the gut microbiome. This is because exposure to a variety of bacteria in the environment helps to diversify the gut microbiome, promoting its health and functionality. To achieve this balance, individuals have adopted a more relaxed approach to hygiene, avoiding the use of antibacterial soaps and excessive use of sanitizers. Instead, they focus on practicing good hygiene practices such as regular handwashing with plain soap and water. Individuals seeking to optimize their microbiome and overall health have made specific changes to their diet and lifestyle. These changes include adopting a plant-based diet, increasing their intake of fermented foods, reducing the use of antibiotics, managing stress levels, prioritizing sleep, and adjusting hygiene routines. By making these changes, individuals are able to promote a healthier and more diverse microbiome, which in turn has a positive impact on their overall health and well-being. Understanding the science of the microbiome and its influence on human health is crucial for achieving optimal nutrition and holistic wellness.

THE HEALTH OUTCOMES THEY ACHIEVED AND HOW THEIR MICROBIOME PLAYED A ROLE

Numerous studies have shown the profound impact that the microbiome has on our overall health and well-being. As individuals began to understand the crucial role that the microbiome plays in their overall health, they took proactive steps to optimize their microbiomes through their diet and lifestyle choices. This deliberate effort led to remarkable health outcomes that have changed their lives for the better.

One of the first health outcomes that individuals achieved through the manipulation of their microbiome was improved digestion. The microbiome is intricately involved in the breakdown and absorption of food in our digestive system. By consuming a diet rich in prebiotic fibers, such as fruits, vegetables, and whole grains, individuals were able to provide their gut microbes with the necessary fuel to thrive. These fibers serve as a food source for beneficial bacteria, enabling them to produce short-chain fatty acids that support optimal digestion. As a result, individuals reported less bloating, improved regularity, and a reduction in gastrointestinal discomfort.

Not only did individuals experience improvements in their digestive health, but they also achieved better immune function through microbiome optimization. The microbiome plays a pivotal role in training and regulating our immune system. By fostering a diverse and balanced microbiome, individuals were able to create an environment that promoted immune tolerance and prevented chronic inflammation.

Immune-related disorders, such as allergies, asthma, and auto-immune conditions, were significantly reduced or even eliminated as a result. This breakthrough in immune health gave individuals greater freedom and relief from the burden of constant sickness and medication management.

Another remarkable health outcome achieved through microbiome manipulation was improved mental health. Recent research has uncovered the powerful connection between the gut and the brain, known as the gut-brain axis. The microbiome produces neurotransmitters, such as serotonin and dopamine, which are essential for regulating mood and emotions. By nourishing their microbiome with a diet rich in probiotics and fermented foods, individuals were able to support the production of these neurotransmitters, leading to a more stable and positive mental state. Anxiety and depression, which had plagued individuals for years, were significantly reduced, allowing them to experience a newfound sense of well-being and emotional balance.

Individuals who optimized their microbiome reported a reduction in chronic inflammation. The gut microbiome has been identified as a key regulator of systemic inflammation throughout the body. By rebalancing their microbiome through dietary interventions, individuals were able to reduce the levels of pro-inflammatory microbes and increase the abundance of anti-inflammatory bacteria. This shift in their gut microbial composition resulted in a decrease in inflammatory markers in their blood, leading to a wide range of health benefits. Notably, individuals experienced relief from chronic pain, improvements in skin conditions such as eczema and acne, and a reduced risk of developing chronic diseases such as cardiovascular disease and diabetes. In addition to these specific health outcomes, individuals who prioritized optimizing their microbiome also reported an overall improvement in their energy levels and vitality. By nourishing their gut bacteria with a diverse range of fibers and polyphenols found in plant-based foods, individuals provided their microbiome with the tools it needs to produce energy efficiently. As a result, individuals experienced a significant reduction in fatigue, increased mental clarity, and improved physical performance. This newfound energy allowed individuals to fully engage in their daily activities and pursue a more active and fulfilling lifestyle. The microbiome plays a critical role in determining our health outcomes, and by understanding its impact, individuals have taken charge of their well-being by manipulating their microbiome through diet and lifestyle choices. The health outcomes achieved have been remarkable, with improvements in digestion, immune function, mental health, inflammation, and energy levels. This newfound understanding of the microbiome and its intervention on our health has revolutionized the concept of optimal nutrition and paved the way for a holistic approach to wellness. As further research continues to unveil the profound impact of the microbiome, individuals are empowered to make informed choices that support their microbiome and ultimately optimize their overall health and vitality.

The human microbiome, consisting of trillions of microorganisms that reside in and on our bodies, plays a significant role in our overall health and well-being. Recent years have seen a surge of research exploring the science of the microbiome and its impact on human health, leading to a deeper understanding of the complex relationship between our gut bacteria and our physical and mental health. It is now widely recognized that the foods we consume have a profound influence on the composition and functioning of our gut microbiota, making optimal nutrition a crucial factor in maintaining a healthy microbiome and promoting holistic wellness. One key area of interest within the study of the microbiome is its role in digestion and nutrient absorption. The gut microbiota, particularly the bacteria that reside in the large intestine, is responsible for breaking down complex carbohydrates and fibers that our own bodies are unable to digest. Through the process of fermentation, these microorganisms produce short-chain fatty acids, such as acetate, propionate, and butyrate, which serve as a vital energy source for our cells. By aiding in the digestion of dietary fiber, the gut microbiota not only contributes to the efficient extraction of nutrients from our food but also plays a crucial role in regulating our metabolism.

In addition to its role in digestion, the microbiome also influences our immune system, mental health, and even our risk of chronic diseases. Researchers have found that a diverse and balanced gut microbiota is associated with a robust immune response and reduced risk of autoimmune disorders. Conversely, an imbalanced microbiome, characterized by a reduction in beneficial bacteria and an overgrowth of harmful bacteria, has been linked to various health issues, including inflammatory bowel diseases, obesity, and even neurological disorders such as depression and anxiety. Given the substantial impact of the microbiome on our health, it is essential to adopt dietary practices that promote a healthy and diverse gut microbiota. One of the most effective ways to do so is by consuming a wide variety of plant-based foods. Fruits, vegetables, whole grains, legumes, and nuts are not only packed with essential vitamins, minerals, and antioxidants but also provide a rich source of dietary fiber. The consumption of dietary fiber has been shown to be strongly associated with a more diverse gut microbiota, as fibers serve as a source of nourishment for beneficial bacteria, helping them thrive and maintain a healthy balance within our gut.

In contrast, a diet high in processed foods, added sugars, and unhealthy fats has been shown to have detrimental effects on the gut microbiome. These types of foods promote the growth of harmful bacteria, leading to an imbalanced microbiota and increased inflammation in the gut. Studies have found that the Western diet, characterized by its high fat and sugar content, can rapidly reduce the diversity of the gut microbiota within a matter of days. Emerging evidence suggests that certain components of our diet, such as the type and amount of protein consumed, can also influence the composition and functioning of the microbiome. For instance, a diet rich in animal-based protein has been associated with a less diverse gut microbiota, while a plant-based diet has been shown to promote a more diverse and favorable microbial profile. These findings highlight the importance of considering not only macronutrient composition but also the source of protein in our diet when aiming to optimize our gut health. As our understanding of the microbiome continues to evolve, so too does the field of nutritional science. Researchers are now exploring the use of prebiotics, probiotics, and even fecal microbiota transplantation as potential interventions to restore a healthy microbiome in individuals with imbalances or disorders. It is important to note that while these interventions show promise, they are not a substitute for a healthy diet and lifestyle. The science of the microbiome has revealed the pivotal role played by our gut bacteria in maintaining our health and well-being. Optimal nutrition, characterized by a varied and plant-based diet, is key to promoting a healthy and diverse microbiome. By consuming foods that support the growth of beneficial bacteria, we can enhance our digestive processes, support a robust immune system, and reduce our risk of chronic diseases. The understanding of the microbiome is a compelling reminder that the foods we choose to fuel our bodies have a profound impact on our overall wellness.

XIII. THE FUTURE OF MICROBIOME RESEARCH AND NUTRITION

As our understanding of the microbiome deepens, it becomes apparent that the field of microbiome research has immense potential for further growth and exploration. There are several key areas that researchers are focusing on in order to unlock the full potential of this exciting field. One area of interest lies in uncovering the role of the microbiome in specific diseases and conditions. By studying the differences in microbiomes between healthy individuals and those afflicted with various diseases, researchers hope to gain insight into the mechanisms by which the microbiome influences our health and wellness.

There has been increasing evidence linking the microbiome to conditions such as obesity, metabolic syndrome, and even mental health disorders. For instance, studies have shown that individuals with obesity have distinct gut microbiomes compared to their lean counterparts, and that the transplantation of gut bacteria from obese individuals into mice can induce weight gain. This suggests a potential role for the microbiome in regulating metabolism and body weight. Similarly, the gut-brain axis, which refers to the bidirectional communication between the gut and the brain, has become an area of intense interest. Emerging research suggests that alterations in the gut microbiome may contribute to the development of mental health disorders such as anxiety and depression. This connection between the gut and the brain opens up new avenues for potential treatment strategies, such as the use of probiotics or prebiotics to modulate the microbiome and improve mental health outcomes. Another area of future research involves the development of personalized nutrition interventions based on an individual's unique microbiome composition. The idea of "one-size-fits-all" diets is being replaced by the concept of personalized nutrition, where dietary recommendations are tailored to an individual's specific microbiome profile. By considering an individual's unique microbial makeup, researchers hope to optimize the nutritional interventions and improve outcomes.

Advancements in technology, particularly in the field of "omics" sciences (genomics, proteomics, metabolomics, etc.) have played a crucial role in pushing the boundaries of microbiome research. These technologies allow for a comprehensive analysis of the microbiome, providing researchers with a wealth of information on microbial composition, function, and interactions. As these techniques become more accessible and affordable, they hold great promise for further advancing our understanding of the microbiome and its impact on human health.

One key challenge in microbiome research lies in deciphering the complex interactions between the microbiome and other factors such as diet, lifestyle, and genetics. The microbiome is highly dynamic and is influenced by a multitude of factors, making it difficult to isolate the effects of individual variables.

Nevertheless, efforts are being made to carefully design experiments and studies that can help disentangle these complex relationships. The future of microbiome research also holds great promise for the development of novel therapeutic strategies. The use of fecal microbiota transplantation (FMT), which involves transferring fecal material containing a healthy microbiome into individuals with certain conditions, has shown remarkable success in treating recurrent Clostridium difficile infection. Researchers are now exploring the potential of FMT for other conditions, such as inflammatory bowel disease, irritable bowel syndrome, and even metabolic disorders.

In addition to FMT, the development of next-generation probiotics and prebiotics is an area of active research. These new formulations aim to target specific microbial species or functions in order to promote a healthy microbiome and improve health outcomes. For example, researchers are investigating the use of engineered probiotics that can deliver therapeutic molecules or modulate specific microbial functions.

The future of microbiome research and nutrition holds incredible promise for improving our health and well-being. By unraveling the intricate relationship between the microbiome and human health, researchers hope to develop personalized nutrition interventions, novel therapeutic strategies, and enhance our overall understanding of human biology. The potential to prevent and treat a wide range of diseases, from obesity and metabolic disorders to mental health conditions, is within our grasp. With continued advancements in technology and dedicated research efforts, we are poised to unlock the full potential of the microbiome for holistic wellness.

CURRENT TRENDS AND ADVANCEMENTS IN MICROBIOME RESEARCH

There has been a growing interest in the field of microbiome research, with numerous advancements and trends emerging. One prominent trend in this field is the focus on the gut microbiome. Researchers have discovered that the gut microbiome plays a crucial role in various aspects of human health, including digestion, metabolism, and immune function. As a result, there is a renewed emphasis on understanding the composition and function of the gut microbiome and how it can be manipulated to improve health outcomes. Advancements in technology have greatly contributed to the progress in microbiome research. DNA sequencing techniques, such as shotgun metagenomics and 16S rRNA sequencing, have enabled researchers to identify and characterize the vast array of microbial species present in different body sites. This has led to a better understanding of the diversity and dynamics of the microbiome and its potential impact on human health. Advances in bioinformatics and computational tools have allowed for the analysis and interpretation of large-scale microbiome data, facilitating the identification of specific microbial taxa or functional genes associated with health or disease states. One of the key findings in microbiome research is the association between gut dysbiosis and various health conditions. Dysbiosis refers to an imbalance or disruption in the gut microbial community, often characterized by a decrease in beneficial bacteria and an overgrowth of potentially harmful microbes. Studies have shown that gut dysbiosis is associated with a wide range of conditions, including inflammatory bowel disease, obesity, type 2 diabetes, and even mental health disorders such as depression and anxiety. This has led to the exploration of therapeutic interventions aimed at restoring a healthy gut microbiome. Probiotics and prebiotics have emerged as popular interventions for promoting a healthy gut microbiome. Probiotics are live microorganisms that, when consumed in adequate amounts, confer a health benefit to the host. These can be found in certain fermented foods or obtained through supplements. Research has shown that probiotics can help restore a disrupted gut microbiome by promoting the growth of beneficial bacteria and inhibiting the growth of pathogenic microbes. Prebiotics, on the other hand, are non-digestible fibers that serve as food for beneficial bacteria in the gut. By selectively feeding these beneficial microbes, prebiotics can help improve the overall composition and function of the gut microbiome. Another current trend in microbiome research is the exploration of the gut-brain axis. The gut and the brain communicate bidirectionally through various pathways, including neural, endocrine, and immune signals. This axis plays a significant role in regulating mood, cognition, and behavior. Research has shown that the gut microbiome can influence brain development and function, and alterations in the gut microbial composition have been associated with psychiatric disorders such as autism spectrum disorder and depression. These findings have led to the emergence of a new field called "psychobiotics," which focuses on using specific strains of bacteria or their metabolites as potential therapies for mental health disorders.

Personalized nutrition has gained traction in the realm of microbiome research. It is now understood that individuals have unique microbial profiles that can influence their response to different dietary interventions. By taking into account an individual's microbiome composition, researchers aim to develop personalized dietary recommendations that can optimize health outcomes. This approach, known as "precision nutrition," holds promise for preventing or managing diseases by tailoring dietary interventions to an individual's specific microbiome.

Recent advancements in microbiome research have shed light on the crucial role of the gut microbiome in human health. The use of advanced sequencing technologies, alongside computational tools and bioinformatics has led to a better understanding of the diversity and dynamics of the microbiome. Dysbiosis has been identified as a common feature of various health conditions, leading to the exploration of interventions such as probiotics and prebiotics to restore a healthy gut microbiome. The gut-brain axis has emerged as a significant area of study, highlighting the bidirectional communication between the gut and the brain. Personalized nutrition has gained momentum, aiming to tailor dietary recommendations to an individual's unique microbiome composition. These trends and advancements in microbiome research hold great potential for improving human health and well-being.

HOW ONGOING DISCOVERIES WILL CONTINUE TO SHAPE OUR UNDERSTANDING OF OPTIMAL NUTRITION

Ongoing discoveries in the field of nutrition research have led to a significant shift in our understanding of what constitutes optimal nutrition. It is now widely recognized that our diets play a crucial role in shaping the composition and diversity of our gut microbiome, which in turn has profound implications for our overall health and well-being. The microbiome refers to the trillions of microorganisms that inhabit our gastrointestinal tract, including bacteria, fungi, and viruses. These microorganisms have a complex and dynamic relationship with the foods we consume, breaking down and fermenting dietary components that our bodies cannot digest on their own. As a result, the microbiome influences key aspects of our physiology, such as metabolism, immune function, and even mental health.

One of the most exciting areas of ongoing research is the exploration of the specific dietary factors that can promote a more beneficial composition of the gut microbiome. For instance, studies have shown that a plant-based diet rich in fiber, fruits, and vegetables can lead to a higher abundance of beneficial bacteria in the gut. These bacteria, such as Bifidobacterium and Lactobacillus, are known for their ability to produce short-chain fatty acids (SCFAs), which provide energy for our gut cells and have anti-inflammatory effects. Conversely, diets high in processed foods and sugar have been associated with a less diverse and less healthy gut microbiome.

Ongoing research is shedding light on the intricate interplay between the gut microbiome and the immune system. It is now understood that the gut microbiome acts as a gatekeeper for our immune system, training it to recognize and respond appropriately to harmful pathogens while tolerating harmless or beneficial microorganisms. This delicate balance can be disrupted by factors such as antibiotic use, which can eliminate both harmful and beneficial bacteria, leading to imbalances in the microbiome and subsequent immune dysregulation. As a result, ongoing research aims to identify dietary strategies that can promote immune health through the cultivation of a diverse and resilient gut microbiome. Another area of ongoing research is the role of the gut microbiome in mental health and well-being. The gut-brain axis, a bidirectional communication network between the gut and the brain, has attracted significant attention in recent years. Studies have found associations between alterations in the gut microbiome and conditions such as anxiety, depression, and autism spectrum disorders. For example, animal studies have shown that altering the gut microbiome composition through probiotic supplementation can affect behavior and mood. Human studies are now starting to explore the potential of modulating the gut microbiome as a novel approach for mental health interventions.

Ongoing discoveries in the field of personalized nutrition have the potential to revolutionize the way we approach dietary recommendations. It is increasingly recognized that individuals respond differently to the same foods, due in part to variations in their gut microbiome. These inter-individual differences can influence our ability to metabolize certain nutrients, the production of SCFAs, and even the potential for weight gain or loss. Ongoing research aims to develop techniques for profiling an individual's gut microbiome to guide personalized dietary recommendations tailored to their specific needs and goals.

Ongoing discoveries are continuing to shape our understanding of optimal nutrition by highlighting the crucial role of the gut microbiome in our overall health and well-being. By recognizing the symbiotic relationship between our diet and our microbiome, researchers have uncovered the potential of dietary interventions to promote a more diverse and beneficial gut microbiome. Ongoing research is uncovering the intricate interplay between the microbiome, the immune system, and mental health, offering novel therapeutic avenues for a range of conditions. The emerging field of personalized nutrition holds the promise of tailoring dietary recommendations to individuals based on their unique gut microbiome composition. As these discoveries continue to emerge, they will undoubtedly play a critical role in shaping our understanding of optimal nutrition and revolutionize our approaches to promoting holistic wellness.

POTENTIAL FUTURE IMPLICATIONS FOR PERSONALIZED MEDICINE AND TREATMENT APPROACHES

As our understanding of the microbiome continues to expand, there is great potential for personalized medicine and treatment approaches in the future. With advancements in technology, we are now able to study and analyze the microbial communities that inhabit our bodies in greater detail. This has led to a growing interest in utilizing this knowledge to develop personalized treatment plans for individuals, based on their unique microbiome composition. By understanding the specific bacteria and other microorganisms present in an individual's gut, for example, healthcare professionals may be able to target treatments more effectively, leading to improved health outcomes. Personalized medicine holds promise for the prevention and management of chronic diseases. Personalized nutrition, in particular, has gained attention as a potential way to optimize health by tailoring dietary recommendations to an individual's unique microbiome. By understanding how different foods interact with the microbiome, personalized nutrition plans may be developed that can support a healthy gut and overall well-being.

One potential implication of personalized medicine is the ability to develop targeted therapeutics based on an individual's microbiome composition. Currently, many medications are designed to have a one-size-fits-all approach, assuming that individuals will respond similarly to treatment. We now know that our microbiomes play a role in drug metabolism, influencing how our bodies respond to medications. By incorporating information about an individual's microbiome into the development of therapeutics, medications could be tailored to maximize their effectiveness and minimize potential side effects. This could revolutionize the field of medicine, allowing for more precise and personalized treatment plans. Personalized medicine may also have a significant impact on the prevention and management of chronic diseases. Chronic conditions, such as obesity, diabetes, and cardiovascular disease, are influenced by a complex interplay between genetic factors, lifestyle choices, and the microbiome. By understanding an individual's genetic predispositions along with their unique microbiome composition, healthcare professionals may be able to identify personalized interventions to prevent the onset or progression of these diseases. For example, certain gut bacteria have been associated with obesity, and by targeting these bacteria, it may be possible to develop interventions that promote weight loss or mitigate the risk of obesity-related complications.

Personalized nutrition is a specific area within personalized medicine that holds great potential for improving health outcomes. The foods we eat have a profound impact on the composition and function of our microbiomes. Tailoring dietary recommendations to an individual's specific microbiome composition may optimize gut health and overall well-being. This concept is known as "precision nutrition" or "nutrigenomics." By sequencing an individual's microbiome and analyzing it for specific microbial markers, healthcare professionals may be able to identify personalized dietary recommendations that can support a healthy gut. For example, if an individual has a low abundance of certain beneficial bacteria, they may be advised to consume more prebiotic-rich foods, such as fruits, vegetables, and whole grains, which can promote the growth of these bacteria. Conversely, individuals with an overgrowth of harmful bacteria may be advised to limit their intake of certain foods that can exacerbate this imbalance, such as highly processed foods or sugary beverages. The expanding field of personalized medicine offers great potential for improving health outcomes and advancing treatment approaches. By incorporating knowledge of an individual's microbiome composition into the development of pharmaceuticals and treatment plans, healthcare professionals may be able to provide more precise and effective interventions. Personalized nutrition holds promise for optimizing health by tailoring dietary recommendations to an individual's unique microbiome. As our understanding of the microbiome continues to deepen, personalized medicine may revolutionize the way we approach health and wellness, leading to more personalized and effective treatment strategies for individuals. The human microbiome is a complex ecosystem that consists of trillions of microorganisms, including bacteria, viruses, fungi, and other microbes, residing in and on our bodies. This remarkable collection of organisms plays a crucial role in maintaining our overall health and well-being. Over the past decade, there has been a growing body of research suggesting that the microbiome is intricately linked to our immune system, metabolism, brain function, and even our mental health. As scientists delve deeper into this fascinating field of study, they are discovering that optimal nutrition is key to maintaining a healthy microbiome and achieving holistic wellness.

The food we consume acts as a fuel for both our bodies and the microbiota that reside within us. Every morsel we eat has the potential to shape the composition and function of our microbiome. Consuming a diet that is rich in diverse plant-based fibers provides the necessary nourishment for the beneficial bacteria in our gut to thrive. These fibers cannot be digested by our own enzymes but are broken down by the bacteria in our colon through a process called fermentation. This fermentation process produces short-chain fatty acids (SCFAs), such as acetate, propionate, and butyrate, which have been shown to have numerous health benefits. Butyrate, in particular, has emerged as a star player in maintaining gut health. It acts as a source of energy for the cells lining our colon, promotes the growth of beneficial bacteria, and has anti-inflammatory properties. Studies have linked low levels of butyrate to various gastrointestinal disorders, such as inflammatory bowel disease and colorectal cancer. A diet rich in butyrate-promoting foods, such as whole grains, legumes, and fruits, can help support a healthy gut environment. In addition to fiber, beneficial bacteria in the gut also require certain nutrients to function optimally. These include prebiotics, which are indigestible carbohydrates that selectively nourish the beneficial bacteria, and probiotics, which are live microorganisms that confer health benefits when consumed in adequate amounts. Prebiotics can be found in foods such as onions, garlic, bananas, and asparagus, while probiotics are abundant in fermented foods like yogurt, sauerkraut, and kimchi. Including these foods in our diet helps to maintain a healthy balance of beneficial bacteria in the gut, which is essential for overall health. But it's not just about the foods we should eat; it's also about the foods we should avoid. Research has shown that diets high in saturated fats, sugar, and processed foods can negatively impact the diversity and function of the microbiome. These dietary patterns have been linked to an increased risk of chronic diseases, including obesity, type 2 diabetes, cardiovascular disease, and certain cancers. A study published in the journal Cell Host & Microbe found that a diet high in saturated fats reduced the diversity of gut bacteria and increased the production of bacterial metabolites that promote inflammation. Another study published in the journal Nature Communications suggested that a diet high in sugar altered the composition of the gut microbiota, leading to increased susceptibility to inflammatory bowel disease. Understanding the intricate relationship between our microbiome and nutrition is essential for optimizing our health. By adopting a diet that supports a diverse and thriving microbiota, we can reap the benefits of enhanced immune function, improved metabolism, and overall holistic wellness. It is worth noting that individual responses to specific dietary interventions may vary, as our microbiomes are as unique as our fingerprints. What works for one person may not work for another. It is important to listen to our bodies and pay attention to the signals they give us. The science of the microbiome has opened up a new frontier in our understanding of human health. The composition and function of our microbiome are influenced by our diet, and in turn, our microbiome has a profound impact on our overall health and well-being. Consuming a diet rich in diverse plant-based fibers, prebiotics, and probiotics, while avoiding diets high in saturated fats, sugar, and processed foods, can help support a healthy and balanced microbiome. By nourishing our microbiome, we can achieve optimal nutrition and holistic wellness for a thriving body and mind.

XIV. CONCLUSION

The microbiome plays a crucial role in our overall health and well-being. Through an intricate symbiotic relationship, the microorganisms in our gut help in the breakdown and absorption of nutrients, modulate our immune system, produce essential vitamins and metabolites, and even communicate with our brain. The composition and diversity of the microbiome are largely influenced by our diet and lifestyle choices, highlighting the significance of nutrition in maintaining a healthy microbiome. A diet rich in fiber, fruits, vegetables, and fermented foods can promote a diverse and balanced microbiome, while a diet high in processed foods and sugar can lead to dysbiosis and inflammation. The use of antibiotics, stress, and lack of physical activity can also negatively impact our microbiome. As our understanding of the microbiome continues to grow, so does the potential for targeted interventions to improve our health. Probiotics, prebiotics, and postbiotics are emerging as key players in microbiome research and may hold promise in the prevention and treatment of various diseases. The concept of personalized nutrition, taking into account an individual's microbiome composition, genetics, and lifestyle factors, is also gaining traction, paving the way for tailored dietary recommendations that can optimize health outcomes. It is important to note that the field of microbiome research is still in its infancy, and much more investigation is needed to fully understand the complex mechanisms at play. Nonetheless, the potential of harnessing the power of the microbiome to improve our health is immense and holds great promise for the future of medicine and nutrition. By appreciating the integral role of our microbiome and making conscious choices to support its health, we can promote holistic wellness and enhance our overall quality of life.

RECAP OF THE IMPORTANCE OF THE MICROBIOME FOR HUMAN HEALTH

The microbiome plays a pivotal role in maintaining our overall health and well-being. This complex ecosystem of bacteria, viruses, fungi, and other microorganisms that reside in our gut has a profound impact on various aspects of our health, including digestion, immune function, mental health, and even weight regulation. Through their interaction with our immune system, these microbes help defend our bodies against harmful pathogens, while also ensuring the proper development and function of our immune system. The microbiome is intricately involved in the breakdown and absorption of nutrients from the foods we consume, thereby influencing our nutritional status. Not only do these microorganisms produce essential vitamins and minerals, but they also ferment dietary fibers to produce short-chain fatty acids, such as butyrate, which have been shown to have anti-inflammatory and protective effects on the colon.

The microbiome has emerged as a key regulator of our mental health and mood. The gut-brain axis, a bidirectional communication network between the gut and the brain, allows for the exchange of signals and molecules, influencing our emotions and cognitive function. Recent research has demonstrated a strong correlation between alterations in the gut microbiota and various mental health disorders, including depression and anxiety. It is believed that these changes in the microbiome can lead to imbalances in neurotransmitter production and inflammation, thereby contributing to the development of mental illness. The microbiome has been implicated in the regulation of body weight and metabolism. Studies have shown that individuals with a healthier and more diverse gut microbiota are less likely to be obese and have a lower risk of developing metabolic disorders such as type 2 diabetes. One mechanism by which the microbiome influences weight is through its ability to extract energy from ingested food. Certain bacteria in the gut are particularly efficient at breaking down complex carbohydrates that our bodies cannot digest, allowing us to extract additional calories from our diet. These microbes can also influence our appetite and food cravings by producing signaling molecules that communicate with our brain. In light of the numerous roles the microbiome plays in our health, it is imperative that we take proactive steps to maintain optimal gut health. One of the most effective ways to support a healthy microbiome is through our diet. Consuming a diverse range of plant-based foods, such as fruits, vegetables, whole grains, legumes, and nuts, provides our gut with a wide array of beneficial fiber and phytochemicals, which act as a fuel source for our gut bacteria. Fermented foods such as yogurt, sauerkraut, and kimchi contain live active cultures of beneficial bacteria, known as probiotics, which can help replenish and diversify the gut microbiota.

It is not only about what we eat but also how we eat. Studies have shown that the way food is processed or cooked can impact the nutritional composition and subsequent effects on the microbiome. For example, excessive heat can destroy certain beneficial compounds and fibers in food, limiting their ability to support the growth of beneficial bacteria in the gut. It is important to prioritize cooking methods that preserve the integrity of these compounds, such as steaming or lightly sautéing vegetables. In addition to diet, lifestyle factors also play a significant role in shaping the microbiome. Chronic stress, lack of sleep, sedentary behavior, and antibiotic use have all been shown to have detrimental effects on the diversity and composition of the gut microbiota. Implementing stress-management techniques, getting adequate sleep, engaging in regular physical activity, and using antibiotics judiciously are all important for maintaining a healthy microbiome. The microbiome is a fascinating and intricate ecosystem that holds immense potential for improving our health and well-being. By understanding the importance of the microbiome and its role in human health, we can make informed decisions about our diet and lifestyle choices to optimize our microbial communities. Through simple yet impactful changes, such as eating a diverse range of plant-based foods, incorporating probiotics into our diet, cooking food in a way that preserves its beneficial compounds, and adopting healthy lifestyle habits, we can support a thriving microbiome and ultimately improve our overall health.

SUMMARY OF THE KEY ASPECTS OF OPTIMAL NUTRITION FOR MICROBIOME HEALTH

Optimal nutrition plays a critical role in supporting the health and well-being of our microbiome. The microbiome refers to the trillions of microorganisms that reside in and on our bodies, particularly within our gut. These microorganisms, which include bacteria, viruses, fungi, and other microbes, play a vital role in various physiological processes and have a profound impact on our overall health. Understanding the key aspects of optimal nutrition for microbiome health is crucial for maintaining holistic wellness. First and foremost, a diverse and balanced diet is essential for promoting a healthy microbiome. Consuming a wide variety of fruits, vegetables, whole grains, legumes, nuts, and seeds provides our microbiome with a range of nutrients and fibers, which serve as fuel for the growth and activity of beneficial bacteria. These beneficial bacteria help to break down and digest complex carbohydrates and fiber that our bodies cannot metabolize alone. Certain types of fiber, known as prebiotics, act as a source of nourishment for beneficial microbes, promoting their growth and enhancing their functionality. Incorporating a variety of plant-based foods into our diets is paramount for supporting a healthy and diverse microbiome.

The quality of the foods we consume greatly influences our microbiome health. Processed foods, rich in added sugars, unhealthy fats, and other artificial additives, have been linked to unfavorable changes in the composition and functioning of the microbiome. Whole, unprocessed foods, such as fruits, vegetables, whole grains, and lean proteins, provide our bodies with essential nutrients and support a diverse and thriving microbiota. These unprocessed foods are also abundant in antioxidants and phytochemicals, which possess anti-inflammatory properties that can positively impact the microbiome. In addition to a diverse and high-quality diet, managing our intake of macronutrients is crucial for maintaining optimal microbiome health. Research has shown that a high-fat diet can lead to an imbalance in the microbiota composition and reduced microbial diversity. Diets rich in healthy fats, such as those found in avocados, olive oil, nuts, and seeds, have been associated with a more favorable microbiome profile. Similarly, excessive consumption of refined carbohydrates, such as white bread and sugary drinks, can disrupt the balance of the microbiome and promote the growth of harmful bacteria. Finding the right balance of macronutrients, including healthy fats, proteins, and complex carbohydrates, is essential for supporting a thriving microbiota. The timing and frequency of our meals can also affect our microbiome health. Recent studies have emphasized the importance of maintaining regular meal patterns and avoiding prolonged periods of fasting. Disruptions in meal timing and prolonged periods of fasting can alter the microbial circadian rhythm, leading to an unfavorable microbiome profile. Incorporating regular eating patterns, avoiding long gaps between meals, and refraining from late-night snacking can help maintain a healthy and balanced gut microbiota.

The impact of certain dietary components, such as probiotics and fermented foods, on the microbiome cannot be overlooked. Probiotics are live microorganisms that, when consumed in adequate amounts, confer health benefits to the host. These beneficial bacteria can be found in foods such as yogurt, kefir, sauerkraut, and kimchi. Consuming probiotic-rich foods can help introduce beneficial bacteria into our gut, enhancing microbial diversity and functionality. Similarly, fermented foods, such as tempeh and miso, contain live bacteria that can positively influence the microbiome. Incorporating these foods into our diet can provide a natural source of beneficial bacteria and contribute to overall gut health. Optimal nutrition plays a critical role in supporting the health and functionality of our microbiome. Consuming a diverse and balanced diet, rich in whole, unprocessed foods, provides our microbiota with the necessary nutrients and fibers to thrive. Managing our intake of macronutrients, maintaining regular meal patterns, and incorporating probiotics and fermented foods also contribute to the health of our microbiome. By understanding and implementing these key aspects of optimal nutrition, we can improve our microbiome health and enhance our overall well-being.

CALL TO ACTION FOR INDIVIDUALS TO PRIORITIZE THEIR MICROBIOME HEALTH THROUGH DIETARY CHOICES

It is clear that the microbiome plays a crucial role in our overall health and well-being. Through its intricate interactions with the immune system, metabolism, and brain, the microbiome has the power to influence various aspects of our health, from digestion and nutrient absorption to mood and mental health. As such, it is imperative that individuals prioritize their microbiome health through dietary choices. By consuming a diet rich in fiber, prebiotics, and probiotics, individuals can promote a diverse and resilient microbiome community, which in turn can support their overall health. Individuals should aim to reduce their consumption of ultra-processed foods, artificial sweeteners, and excessive antibiotic use, as these have been shown to negatively impact the diversity and composition of the microbiome. Engaging in regular physical activity, managing stress levels, and getting enough sleep are also important factors in maintaining a healthy microbiome. Individuals should be mindful of the potential long-term consequences of their dietary choices on their microbiome health. The decisions we make today can have a profound impact on the health of our microbiome, and in turn, our overall well-being. It is essential that we prioritize our microbiome health and make informed dietary choices for optimal nutrition and holistic wellness. With further research and understanding of the microbiome, we can continue to uncover the intricate connections between our diet, microbiome, and health, ultimately paving the way for personalized nutrition recommendations. By harnessing the power of our microbiome, we can optimize our health and potentially prevent or mitigate the risk of various diseases. The time to prioritize our microbiome health is now, as the benefits extend far beyond our digestive system. So, let us come together and embrace the call to action for individuals to prioritize their microbiome health through dietary choices. Making mindful and informed decisions about the foods we consume can have a tremendous impact on our overall health and well-being. By nourishing our microbiome with the right foods, we can ensure that it thrives and supports our body in various ways. Let us choose a diverse and plant-based diet, rich in fiber, prebiotics, and probiotics, to nurture our microbiome and promote optimal health. Let us reduce our reliance on ultra-processed foods and artificial sweeteners, which have been shown to disrupt the delicate balance of our microbiome. Let us be judicious with our use of antibiotics, recognizing their potential consequences on our microbiome health. Let us prioritize regular physical activity, stress management, and quality sleep, as these factors can also influence the composition and function of our microbiome. And above all, let us remember that the choices we make today can have a lasting impact on our microbiome health and overall well-being. So, take the call to action and prioritize your microbiome health through your dietary choices. Your microbiome will thank you, and your body will too. The microbiome refers to the diverse community of microorganisms that reside in and on the human body. These microorganisms include bacteria, viruses, fungi, and protozoa, and they play a crucial role in maintaining our health. The human microbiome is thought to contain around 100 trillion microbial cells, outnumbering human cells by a factor of ten. Recent research has shown that the microbiome is not only important for digestion and nutrient absorption but also for overall health and well-being. The microbiome has been linked to a variety of conditions, including obesity, diabetes, autoimmune diseases, and mental health disorders. One of the key factors that influence the composition and functioning of the microbiome is diet. The foods we eat can have a profound impact on the types and abundance of microorganisms that reside in our gut. For example, a diet high in fiber has been shown to promote the growth of beneficial bacteria in the gut, while a diet high in saturated fat and sugar can lead to an increase in harmful bacteria. In addition, certain types of food can directly affect the production of short-chain fatty acids, which are compounds produced by gut bacteria that have been linked to numerous health benefits. There has been growing interest in the concept of personalized nutrition, which aims to optimize the diet to an individual's unique microbiome. This approach recognizes that each person's microbiome is different and that what works for one person may not work for another. By understanding the composition of an individual's microbiome, it may be possible to recommend specific dietary interventions that can improve health outcomes. One emerging area of research in the field of microbiome science is the use of prebiotics and probiotics to improve gut health. Prebiotics are indigestible fibers that promote the growth of beneficial bacteria in the gut, while probiotics are live microorganisms that confer health benefits when consumed. These products can be found in a variety of foods, such as yogurt, kefir, sauerkraut, and kimchi. While the effects of prebiotics and probiotics on the microbiome are still being studied, early research suggests that they may have the potential to improve digestion, boost the immune system, and reduce the risk of certain diseases. It is also important to note that the impact of diet on the microbiome is not limited to the gut. Research has shown that the oral microbiome, which consists of bacteria and other microorganisms in the mouth, can also be influenced by diet. For example, a diet high in sugar and processed foods can promote the growth of harmful bacteria in the mouth, leading to dental cavities and gum disease. A diet rich in fruits, vegetables, and whole grains can promote the growth of beneficial bacteria in the oral microbiome, contributing to oral health. The microbiome is a complex and fascinating ecosystem that plays a crucial role in human health. Diet is a major factor that influences the composition and functioning of the microbiome, with certain foods promoting the growth of beneficial bacteria, while others can lead to an increase in harmful bacteria. Personalized nutrition, prebiotics, and probiotics offer promising ways to optimize the microbiome for improved health outcomes. It is important to recognize that the impact of diet on the microbiome is not limited to the gut but also extends to other areas of the body, such as the oral microbiome. By understanding the science of the microbiome and its relationship with nutrition, we can make informed dietary choices that promote holistic wellness and improve our overall health.

BIBLIOGRAPHY

Pankaj Bhatt. 'Recent Advancements in Microbial Diversity.' Surajit de Mandal, Academic Press, 6/2/2020

Jeannette Hyde. 'The Gut Makeover.' 4 Weeks to Nourish Your Gut, Revolutionize Your Health, and Lose Weight, Bloomsbury Publishing, 5/2/2017

Sergio Rijo. 'Defying Age.' The Ultimate Guide to Living a Long and Healthy Life, SERGIO RIJO, 4/10/2023

Institute of Medicine. 'U.S. Health in International Perspective.' Shorter Lives, Poorer Health, National Research Council, National Academies Press, 4/12/2013

Damian J. Anderson. 'Gut First, Health Follows.' A Holistic Approach to Healing the Gut Microbiome, UNLYN, 4/15/2023

Health and Medicine Division. 'Nutrigenomics and the Future of Nutrition.' Proceedings of a Workshop, National Academies of Sciences, Engineering, and Medicine, National Academies Press, 8/27/2018

Lynnette R. Ferguson. 'Nutrigenomics and Nutrigenetics in Functional Foods and Personalized Nutrition.' CRC Press, 4/19/2016

Tomas Hajek. 'Brain-Metabolic Crossroads in Severe Mental Disorders – Focus on Metabolic Syndrome.' Virginio Salvi, Frontiers Media SA, 10/23/2019

Adrien A Eshraghi. 'Gut-brain Connection, Myth Or Reality?: Role Of The Microbiome In Health And Diseases.' World Scientific, 11/3/2021

Martin J. Blaser, MD. 'Missing Microbes.' How the Overuse of Antibiotics Is Fueling Our Modern Plagues, Henry Holt and Company, 4/8/2014

Will Bulsiewicz, MD. 'Fiber Fueled.' The Plant-Based Gut Health Program for Losing Weight, Restoring Your Health, and Optimizing Your Microbiome, Penguin, 5/12/2020

World Health Organization. 'Guideline: Sugars Intake for Adults and Children.' World Health Organization, 3/31/2015

Madiha M. Saeed MD. 'The Holistic Rx.' Your Guide to Healing Chronic Inflammation and Disease, Rowman & Littlefield, 10/13/2017

C. Senaka Ranadheera. 'Probiotics and Prebiotics in Foods.' Challenges, Innovations, and Advances, Adriano Gomes da Cruz, Academic Press, 3/23/2021

Victor R Preedy. 'Probiotics, Prebiotics, and Synbiotics.' Bioactive Foods in Health Promotion, Ronald Ross Watson, Academic Press, 9/23/2015

Raphael Kellman. 'Microbiome Diet.' The Scientifically Proven Way to Restore Your Gut Health and Achieve Permanent Weight Loss, Hachette Books, 7/1/2014

Samuli Rautava. 'The Human Microbiome in Early Life.' Implications to Health and Disease, Omry Koren, Academic Press, 9/18/2020

Dirk Haller. 'The Gut Microbiome in Health and Disease.' Springer, 7/27/2018

Pallaval Veera Bramhachari. 'Microbiome in Human Health and Disease.' Springer Nature, 10/18/2021

Division on Earth and Life Studies. 'Environmental Chemicals, the Human Microbiome, and Health Risk.' A Research Strategy, National Academies of Sciences, Engineering, and Medicine, National Academies Press, 3/1/2018

Angela E. Douglas. 'Fundamentals of Microbiome Science.' How Microbes Shape Animal Biology, Princeton University Press, 6/8/2021

Food and Nutrition Board. 'The Human Microbiome, Diet, and Health.' Workshop Summary, Food Forum, National Academies Press, 2/27/2013